beautiful selling

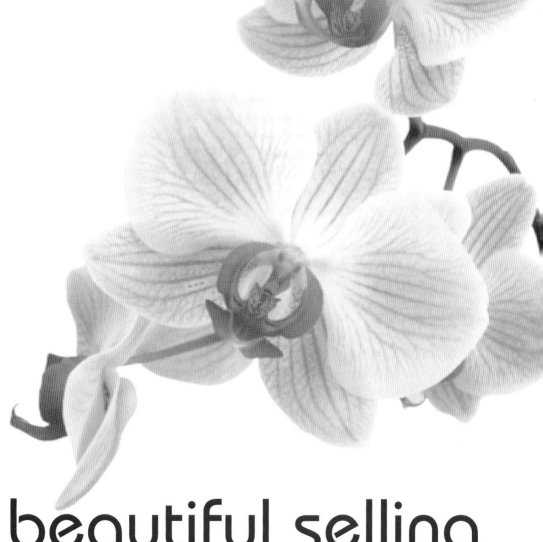

beautiful selling

ruth langley

the complete guide to sales success in the salon

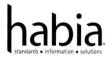

standards • information • solutions

City&
Guilds

THOMSON™

Australia • Canada • Mexico • Singapore • Spain • United Kingdom • United States

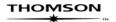

THOMSON
™

beautiful selling
the complete guide to sales success in the salon
ruth langley

Publishing Director John Yates	**Commissioning Editor** Melody Woollard	**Development Editor** Alice Rodgers
Content Project Editor Alison Walters	**Manufacturing Manager** Helen Mason	**Marketing Manager** Jason Bennett
Editorial Assistant Matthew Lane	**Production Controller** Maeve Healy	**Cover Design** hctcreative ltd, Hants
Text Design Design Deluxe, Bath	**Printer** G. Canale & C.S.p.A., Italy	**Typesetter** Saxon Graphics Ltd

British Library Cataloguing-in-Publication Data
A catalogue record for this book is available from the British Library

To Harry
With Love

contents

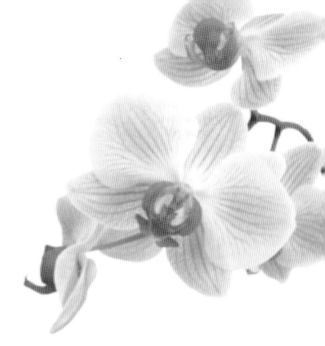

chapter one
what is selling?   1

chapter two
getting your mind ready to sell   12

chapter three
selling yourself 22

chapter four
relationship selling 36

chapter five
the consultation 46

chapter six
product demonstration and presentation 64

chapter seven
product knowledge   84

chapter eight
overcoming objections   102

chapter nine
closing the sale   116

chapter ten
techniques and aids to help you sell   126

chapter eleven
promotions to increase retail sales   134

chapter twelve
goal setting in selling   144

chapter thirteen
creating a sales culture in the salon   156

chapter fourteen
...and finally   170

about the author

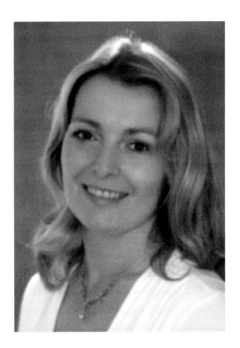

Ruth Langley is a national award winning salon director with over twenty years' hands on experience within the Hair & Beauty industries. As a qualified teacher and life coach, Ruth has a passion for developing therapists' and hairdressers' professional skills in order to deliver first class customer satisfaction. Now viewed as one of the best salon directors in the UK, *Grazia* magazine listed her salon, *Pink Orchid*, as one of the 'Secret A-List Addresses' for luxury new hair treatments.

acknowledgements

Thank you to my husband, Andrew Langley, who has spent a lot of time and effort giving his advice and considerable talent to help develop my career as a sales trainer, author and business consultant. His unwavering belief in me and support has given me the confidence to pursue my goals. In addition, I would like to acknowledge my husband's company, LPS creative media, for the excellent professional photographs provided for this book.

I would like to thank Andrew Leigh of Pathways life coaching for his professional help that guided me in the initial writing of this book. My ideas for the book were turned into reality by his excellent motivational skills and first-class coaching.

Thanks to my parents for their constant love and support in my career and life, they are my 'role models'.

Finally, I would like to thank Thomson Learning, especially Alice and Melody, for the opportunity to publish this book; it has been such a pleasure to do business with them.

preface

Welcome to *Beautiful Selling* and thank you for purchasing this book. I love selling! Yes you read it right: I love selling! My aim is for you, the reader, to feel the same way, to develop the passion and the motivation to increase your retail sales.

Selling is the ultimate profession, each day providing new opportunities to help and advise clients, plus new challenges and unlimited financial rewards.

Opportunities to achieve sales are all around us. Once you have mastered some great sales techniques your confidence levels, motivation and passion for selling will grow. Motivation is clarity and planning, knowing what you want and how you will go about achieving it. *Beautiful Selling* will help show you the way to achieve more sales more of the time and have fun in the process.

> IT IS TIME TO CHANGE THE WAY YOU SEE SELLING …
>
> IT IS TIME TO CHANGE THE WAY YOU FEEL ABOUT SELLING …
>
> NOW IS THE TIME TO BEGIN …
>
> BEAUTIFUL SELLING!

Why I wrote this book

Over the years I have attended sales seminars and read many books on the subject of selling and, whilst I learned many great techniques, I always found much of the information difficult to apply within the salon or spa. For example, how vital it is to keep your clients' interest during the sales process. Now as important as this technique may be, it is pretty difficult to implement when clients are laid on a couch in a deep state of relaxation or even asleep!

My aim with *Beautiful Selling* is to examine the sales process exclusively within the salon and to share with you, the therapist, some effective sales techniques. Many sales books focus heavily on marketing and whilst I agree the two are linked, I passionately believe selling is a skill and profession all of its own.

There are many skills that lead to successful selling, some you may have mastered, others you may wish to develop. *Beautiful Selling* is here to help you. It has been designed to 'fast track' the inexperienced or beginner to sell. It will also act as a reference guide to the more experienced sales person. A single idea can dramatically improve your sales' levels and great success can be achieved from the smallest single idea. One of my all time favourite quotes is from Mr Walt Disney. When referring to his immense success and achievements Disney said:

> 'I only hope that we never lose sight of one thing – that it was all started by a mouse.'

If your do the same things in the same way you will get the same results. *Beautiful Selling* will show and help you change what you are doing to achieve the results you desire.

My promise to you

This book provides knowledge, but knowledge is not power, it is only potential power. YOU need to take action to get the results. Let me explain what I can do for you. I will make selling easier, the sales process clearer and selling more enjoyable. I can help you change the way you think about selling, to view it positively and as a challenge.

I will share with you techniques to close more sales and skills to put you in the top 10 per cent of salespeople in our profession. BUT it all starts with YOU, all I ask is you study these techniques then apply them, in other words TAKE ACTION. Selling is not a spectator sport, this book is not armchair selling, sales success is achieved by taking small consistent steps each and every day to reach your target.

together let's build a sales culture
into your salon

together let's achieve great retail
sales

I believe every therapist has the potential to become a great salesperson.

Ruth Langley

foreword

Selling can provoke negative emotions in all of us. This often stems from experiences where we have felt bullied into purchasing products we don't want.

However, with the hair and beauty product industry booming, it is a big mistake for salons to believe that clients do not want to buy products. In fact, I think it is fair to say that some clients wish they were advised on the benefits of products which would suit them.

Beautiful Selling shows you how to deliver the type of selling your clients want, that which meets clients' needs. Author Ruth Langley has always had her eye focused on the customer in this way.

Ruth Langley has worked for many years as a therapist and salon owner. She has many other strings to her bow including being a qualified teacher, a life coach and a consultant for Habia. She is extremely dynamic and her energy and attention to detail is impressive.

This book is so motivating that it is easy to see why Ruth is a life coach. Following this book will motivate and inspire you and heighten your interpersonal communication and non verbal skills and awareness. What more could you ask for?

Alan Goldsbro
Habia CEO

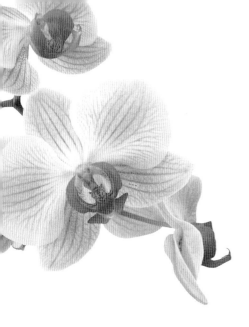

chapter one
what is selling?

Introduction

Selling is the professional recommendation of products to your clients. It is a process where we, the therapist, select the most suitable products for our clients to use at home. Selling is encouraging your clients to adopt an effective home-care routine.

The process of selling can begin through educating your clients. This education technique will help you tremendously, especially if your sales are low due to a fear of selling. Use your expertise to explain, for example, the importance of skin exfoliation and how much your clients' skin will benefit from this. Next, show your clients a suitable product and then demonstrate how to use it. These two simple steps will educate your clients on the importance of skin exfoliation.

you will learn

Within this chapter we will review:

- What selling actually is
- The importance of retailing as a salon service

 tip

Educated clients are more likely to buy.

What is selling?

When you sell you are:

- giving expert advice to your clients
- identifying and meeting your clients' needs
- solving your clients' concerns or problems
- taking the time to care about your clients' home-care routine

- ensuring your clients achieve the results they desire

- helping your clients buy.

In other words, you are offering a great service to your clients.

As beauty therapists we naturally have a caring nature towards our clients. This quality is a great backbone to becoming a successful salesperson.

Selling is a skill. Salespeople are not born, they are made. Whilst it may be true certain personality types make more effective salespeople, all of us have the potential to develop characteristics to become effective at selling.

successful salespeople have:

- a passionate belief that they are helping their clients

- great customer care skills

- a talent of building excellent relationships with their clients

- an ability to see things from their clients' point of view

- an excellent way of transferring passion and enthusiasm of products to clients.

When you introduce a new treatment into your salon, you undergo intensive training to be able to perform it correctly and effectively. The same is true with selling. In order to be good at selling you have to study selling. Selling is a skill and as such needs to be studied then practised until you develop it to an excellent and effective standard.

The more you practise selling the more comfortable, confident and effective you will become.

This book provides the theory, but selling is a skill that you must practise in order to become competent.

the key is to keep going; there is no failure in selling just feedback

I remember my first electrolysis lesson at college. With my hand shaking I inserted the probe and it bent. The skin bled and caused discomfort to my fellow therapist whose follicle I was treating. Although the outcome was not ideal and did not give results, I kept trying. Not only did I pass all my examinations, but I went on to teach electrolysis and develop a life-long love of the treatment. Many of us have experienced failures in selling – lots of bent probes – and therefore tend to shy away from selling. The most successful people have had their failures along their path to riches. However, they kept focused and developed a determination to succeed.

Many of us are great salespeople already we are just not aware of it. As busy therapists we have already sold our unique services to our clients who come back regularly for treatments. Therefore, YOU ARE A GREAT SALESPERSON, you are liked and trusted by your clients. Being liked and trusted are two key characteristics adopted by successful salespeople. All we need to do now is transfer these techniques to retailing products. We are successful treatment providers, now we have to become excellent product providers.

When I studied for my professional certificate in life coaching a key element was common sense. The same key element can be applied with regard to selling. Knowing which questions to ask, when to sell, the right time to close the sale,

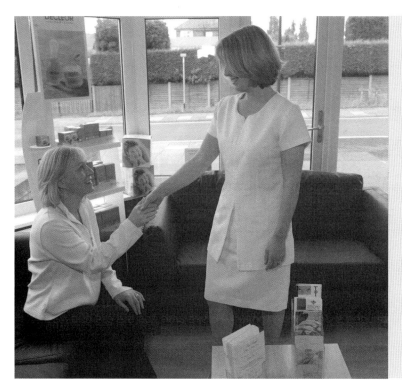

Successful salespeople have great customer care skills

are all examples that require a little common sense, not some amazing magic formula we have yet to discover.

The wheel of selling

The diagram below shows the wheel of selling. This introduces the key principles and ingredients required to develop successful sales.

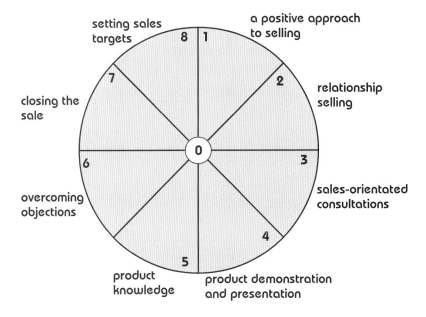

Each area shown on the wheel of selling has an essential role and indeed is vital to the sales process. Let's relate it to baking a cake. To do this successfully, you need certain ingredients: flour, eggs, sugar and butter. If you were to omit one vital ingredient, for example the flour, the cake would not quite be as desired.

Now relate this to selling. Each ingredient on the wheel of selling is vital to your overall performance and the long-term success of your sales career.

The eight ingredients

The wheel of selling diagram introduces you to each stage or part of the sales process.

1 A positive approach to selling

This is the first and probably one of the most important parts of professional selling. You must enjoy selling; view it as a extension of the service you currently offer. Selling is an essential salon service and you are the most qualified person to give advice and product recommendations to your clients.

2 Relationship selling

At the heart of every sale are your clients: their needs are paramount. The most successful salespeople in our industry have an ability to form good client relationships and focus on giving excellent customer care to all their clients.

3 Sales-orientated consultations

Effective consultations are an essential ingredient for selling. Uncovering your clients' needs is an area in which each of us must become skilled and proficient. We need to develop appropriate questions and adopt excellent listening skills.

4 Product demonstration and presentation

It is essential that you can professionally carry out an effective presentation of the products you are recommending to your clients. The demonstration should be informative, educational and tailored exactly to each client's needs.

5 Product knowledge

In order to sell products, you first need to know all about them. A professional salesperson understands the features and benefits of each and every product they sell. They know exactly the results each product can deliver and can transfer this passion to their clients. Product knowledge, in my opinion and experience, is, and always will be, one of the corner stones to successful selling.

6 Overcoming objections

Even the most experienced sales professionals will receive objections when they sell; it is par for the course. What is essential is the ability to handle these objections professionally and confidently.

7 Closing the sale

This is a natural progression in the sales process. Simply asking for the sale is perhaps one of the easiest and quickest parts in selling.

8 Setting sales targets

Anyone serious about selling will constantly be aiming at set sales targets. Targets can motivate and develop your sales career at a rapid rate. They can be daily, weekly, monthly or yearly targets, but a sales goal will keep you on track to success.

Each area will be looked at in much greater depth throughout this book. It is essential to understand though, that each stage on the wheel of selling plays an important part in the sales process. To sell professionally you have to follow a structure or a recipe; let's go back to our cake again. Firstly, you need the right ingredients – flour, eggs, sugar and butter – but secondly, they need to be used in the right order. I presume in most recipes, if you do not use the ingredients in the correct order the end result may not be the original desired outcome. Relate this back to selling: if deep down you do not enjoy selling and you do not passionately believe you are helping your clients, you may find it difficult to close the sale or develop high levels of retail sales.

The wheel of selling was designed for you to see the whole picture of selling and for you the reader to look carefully at each stage and understand which areas are your strengths and which may need some development.

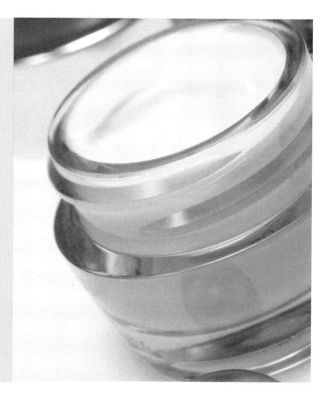

Product knowledge is one of the cornerstones to successful selling

Why retail?

Do you care about your clients?

Do you care enough to perform the best treatments using the best products when they visit the salon?

Do you exceed their expectations?

Are they satisfied and happy clients?

I should guess you have answered yes to all the above questions, now pause and just think for a moment.

How long is each client's treatment?

How much time is spent in your salon?

The reality is that on average clients probably spend between one and two hours each week or month in the salon.

What happens the rest of the time?

What products do they use at home?

Your clients need a home-care routine. Your care should extend to provide this.

> As beauty therapists I believe it is our professional duty to give our clients the best possible recommendations on home-care products and advise on how to correctly use their products at home.

Nowadays clients are better educated about products and if they are not buying them from you then they are purchasing them from someone else.

 tip

If you require a little push to start selling, think about the following scenario:

One of your clients has just enjoyed a facial treatment with you, her professional therapist. After her treatment she leaves the salon and goes directly to a store to purchase her skin care. Why? Simply because she views you as a treatment-only provider and all the advertising done by the large skin-care houses has led her to believe they will provide the products. After all her therapist has never attempted to sell her any products or indeed give her advice.

Who is getting your sales?

Next time you visit a large store, go and observe the staff at skin-care counters at work. Just watch how many products they sell. This experience was motivation enough for me to start selling to my clients. As therapists we have the training, the professional knowledge and the experience – let's start using it. Remember, if you don't seize the opportunity to sell to your clients someone else will.

Create the space to sell. Do not be too busy to sell; it should be part and parcel of the professional service you offer. Expecting clients to buy from you and knowing that clients want to buy products from you are amazing positive beliefs and affirmations to have. Now is the time to remove those negative and limiting beliefs which say 'my clients do not buy from me, they just come to me for their treatments, I feel uncomfortable selling to them'. Go and visit that store again. The salespeople their do not feel uncomfortable, they are helping people buy.

You know, people really enjoy spending, the term 'retail therapy' should re-enforce this point. We all love to buy; our clients have a desire to purchase new products. Do not feel guilty about selling, customers do not feel guilty about buying.

The skin-care industry is a multi-billion pound business in the UK. As beauty therapists let's lead the way to gain the sales that are rightfully ours.

let's start selling!

real life example

my first ever sale

In 1985 I opened my first beauty salon, a small room within a hairdressing salon.

Back in those days the beauty industry was not as popular as it is today, but I was on a personal mission to change all of that. I worked tirelessly to build a clientèle and establish a business. Right from the beginning, however, I had a passion to sell. My parents were in the retail trade and I had virtually been raised in a newsagents shop. From a very early age I would serve customers in the family business, so my exposure to selling goods became natural and normal to me.

Now back to me and my 'little room'; it was harder in those days to encourage clients to have skin treatments let alone purchase products. I had a small selection of retail products, 20 to be exact, all beautifully displayed on three shelves. Each day I would dust and rearrange them and observe how 'lovely' they looked all in their place and all sitting pretty on their shelf. One day, after returning from my lunch break, I entered my beauty room and got a terrible shock … a product was missing. I did a quick count; only 19 products … yes I was right … one had gone … it had been stolen. I raced through to the reception and informed the receptionist what had happened.

Her reply gave me a second shock. She informed me a client that I had treated the previous day had come into the salon to purchase it; apparently I had recommended it during her treatment.

To this day I can still remember my response to the receptionist: 'you mean she came in and actually bought it?' After the shock had subsided, I had an amazing feeling of achievement and I knew from that day forward SELLING would always play a major role in my career.

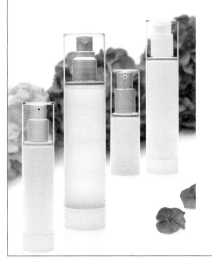

Selling should be part and parcel of the professional service you offer

✔ **key** reminders

- Selling is taking the time to care about your clients' home-care routine.

- Selling is a skill, it has to be studied and practised.

- Successful salespeople have a great ability to transfer their product passion and enthusiasm to their clients.

- Create time to sell – do not be too busy to be successful.

- Your clients need a home-care routine – make sure you are the one who provides it.

Exercises

1 The average client spends one to two hours per month in the salon. Your client will be using products at home. If they are not being purchased from you, then where could your clients be buying them from? List five places:

a

b

c

d

e

2 a What do you feel is the main reason you are not currently selling to your full potential?

b If you could do one thing right now to rectify this, what would it be?

If you don't sell to your clients then someone else will

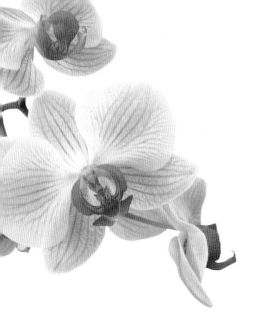

chapter two

getting your mind
ready to sell

Introduction

As I mentioned in the previous chapter, having a positive approach to selling is perhaps one of the most important characteristics you need. The ability to look forward to recommending, advising and selling products to your clients is a step towards creating a perfect positive perspective on selling.

To some people the word 'selling' automatically triggers panic or fear yet selling is not a dirty word. Public speaking is another area where people feel unable to perform. Just the idea of standing up in front of a large group of people fills them with dread. To overcome this fear, I was also told to imagine you are having a conversation with just one person in the audience as oppose to at least 50 people. Within selling, the best advice is to imagine you are simply helping your clients with their home-care. As I said previously I love selling, I am a salesperson and I am proud of it. Each and every day I have the opportunity to offer advice to my clients, help solve their concerns and earn unlimited financial rewards through selling. Each day provides amazing circumstances to achieve more sales and meet challenges with positive expectations. What a great profession!

you will learn

Within this chapter we will review:

- How you think and feel about selling will have a direct impact on your sales levels
- How a positive approach to selling will lead to a positive result

---

- If you believe you are a poor salesperson or a great salesperson you are probably right.
- Your mind is a very powerful tool; your thoughts control your actions.

Getting ready to sell

Each sales process needs you. It needs you to have a positive perspective on selling, so together let's get you and your mind ready to sell. If you fear selling then I have some really good news for you … It is not that bad, in fact the worst outcome I have ever experienced is that my clients may say 'no thank you', that is it. Nothing else will happen, just three little words – no thank you.

In fact selling can be great fun, very rewarding and in addition is quite easy to do once you have mastered the techniques. During each day at the salon, when I get an opportunity to create sales I feel empowered and motivated. I almost get a 'buzz' as it gives me an exciting opportunity to help someone. By adopting this positive perspective you too will welcome sales opportunities and look forward to selling whilst enjoying the whole process.

Customer care is an area where we all strive for excellence. We love to talk about and practice new techniques and very few therapists will have a fear of attempting good customer care. With customer care, however, if you get it wrong you may run a real chance of losing clients. However, when selling, if the sale is not successful it will not have a negative impact on your clients' perception of you. As long as you do not employ any pressure or 'hard sell' techniques, your clients will simply choose not to buy but will still re-book their next treatments as usual and you will not have jeopardized your relationship with them. Here is the good news; during their next visit you can begin the sales process again. With customer care you never get a second chance but with selling you get a second, third, fourth chance and so on.

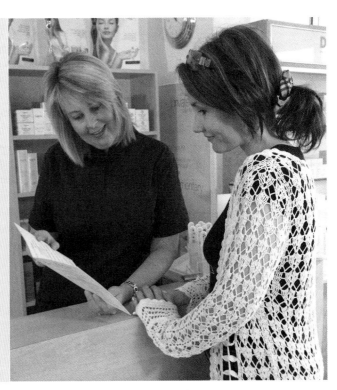

If the sale is not successful it will not reflect badly on you

Learn to love selling

It is time to begin a new chapter in selling. You are the author of your own life so let's write in some sales success, starting with positive expectations. Confidence comes from knowing you are doing the best for your clients combined with the passion and belief in what you are selling. Move out of your comfort zone; aim to stretch your abilities and new-found knowledge to develop higher retail sales. Remember, there are no failures just feedback, each lost sale is a learning opportunity to develop more effective selling skills.

let's get confident!

People who feel good about themselves produce good results. When selling, how you feel about yourself can have a direct impact on the results you achieve.

Below is a selection of ideas to help put you in the right frame of mind.

- You are representing the beauty therapy industry, be proud of this.

- Always work to a high standard of professional ethics.

- Make a commitment to always do your best.

- Your attitude determines your results.

- Your reward will be in direct proportion to your contribution.

- Always respect yourself.

- Always believe in yourself.

- By committing to success and improving yourself, you are on your way to reaching your full potential.

- The more energy you have the more powerful you become.

- Be ahead of the game. The beauty industry is advancing at a rapid rate; change is out there, it is happening. People are investing their time and money on treatments and products, be ready to serve them well and to sell to them well.

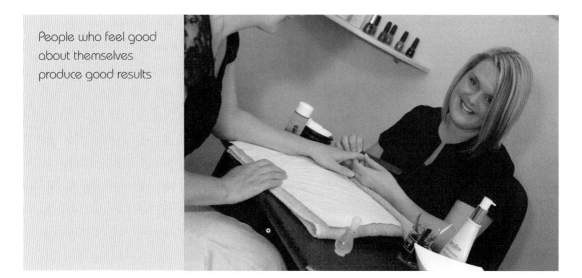

People who feel good
about themselves
produce good results

The power of visualization to help you sell

We all have the ability to create positive images in our minds, pictures which provoke great feelings or happy memories. Try this experiment now:

1 Think of a recent happy event, maybe it was a really good night out with friends, or maybe a particular holiday you went on where you had a really good time.

2 When you think about this special time, how does it make you feel?

As you answer the questions no doubt you will have created images or pictures in your mind of the particular event. You will have accessed your imagination and this in turn will have created wonderful feelings within you. The good news is that we can use our imagination to create positive images and feelings of events that have yet to happen.

I will now share with you a technique which will help you create positive expectations when selling. Before you are about to sell or indeed perform a product demonstration, try this quick simple exercise.

Step 1

Think of yourself as the best qualified person to sell to your client. See yourself as a successful salesperson.

Step 2

Now say to yourself: 'I love selling, I have the knowledge and experience to help people purchase the right products. Clients want me to help them, they look to me for the best solution for homecare advice and they want to buy from me.'

Step 3

Now close your eyes and see your clients buying the products you have recommended, see your clients smiling, happy that someone has taken the time to care.

Step 4

As you run this image through your mind, experience the wonderful feelings and hold on to them. Feel that amazing sense of achievement and self-fulfilment.

You can access these feelings whenever you are getting ready to sell and within time your sales techniques combined with the power of positive visualization will help develop your true sales potential.

✔ key reminders

- Developing a positive approach to selling is a vital ingredient in achieving high retail sales.
- Be proud to be called a salesperson: you are taking the extra time to care about your clients' home-care needs.
- The worst outcome of any sale are the three little words, 'no thank you'.
- When you serve well you will sell well.

real life example

when is the easiest time to make a sale?

The answer to this question is very straight-forward. The easiest time to create a sale is straight after you have just made one. Allow me to give two examples to explain exactly what I mean by this statement.

example 1

My first client of the day listens to the home-care advice I give but decides not to purchase.

My second client of the day does the same.

My third client, after listening to my rec-ommendations, also decides not to pur-chase anything.

By the time my fourth client enters the salon, I do not exactly feel like recommend-ing products or even trying to sell anything. I have lost my enthusiasm.

example 2

My first client loves the advice I have given them and chooses to purchase a cleanser, toner and mask.

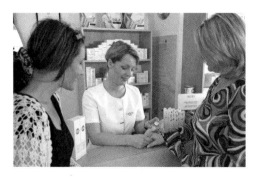

My next client also purchases products.

My third client thinks their skin looks so wonderful after their treatment and asks what products they could use at home and then buys them.

By the time my fourth client is being treated, I am expecting them to buy!

Many therapists will be able to identify with the above examples. In example two, you have 'positive expectations' that each client will buy from you. You will be moti-vated, focused and full of self-confidence. You will be driven by your previous results, your success so far. You will be positive and determined to sell.

The second example is one which I relate to. When I make a sale I seem to 'be on a roll', I become unstoppable! Next time you are in the salon observe either yourself or another therapist once they have sold a product – the chances are they will keep selling.

the motto?

start your day in a selling way!

Think of yourself as the best qualified person to sell to your client because you are.

Exercises

Sales award

Imagine you are receiving an award in recognition of your high level of sales. Over the past 12 months you have sold more products than any other therapist. At the Annual General Meeting an award presentation is being held by your skin-care supplier to recognize your achievement.

As the Managing Director announces your name you walk onto the stage to a standing ovation.

- How would you feel?

- Would you feel proud of your achievement?

- Maybe you would have a great sense of self-fulfilment, because through sheer hard work and determination you have reached your sales potential.

Now, close your eyes and through the power of visualization, run this event through your mind.

Imagine all those empowering feelings, see yourself accepting the award – see yourself as a successful salesperson … because soon you will be.

More sales are lost because they were never asked for

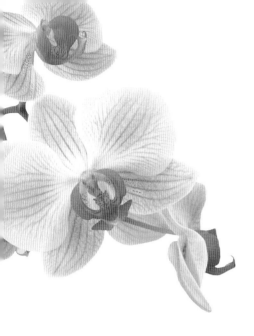

chapter three
selling yourself

Introduction

The first and most important sale you will make is yourself. People tend to buy from someone they like and trust. Never ever forget this. Many therapists are regularly requested by the same clients for treatments and these clients will have been 'regular clients' for many years. There are many reasons why clients insist on visiting the same therapist for each appointment:

- The therapist always performs treatments to a high standard.

- The therapist offers evening and weekend appointments and will always try to accommodate their clients.

- The therapist always gives good advice.

- A complete consultation is performed prior to each treatment to ensure that clients' needs are being met.

The list is endless!

However, the first and most important reason that clients will choose a certain therapist and then continually request them, is that they like them, they get on with them.

It is therefore essential to build a good relationship with your clients in order to achieve great sales.

you will learn

Within this chapter we will review:

- The qualities of successful salespeople
- Developing skills that will enhance your sales performance

 tip

Clients will tend to buy from a therapist they like and trust.

real life example

you can't win them all

As therapists we have an ability to get on well with most people, in fact it is almost a prerequisite of our profession. As a rule, regardless of personality type, we find it both natural and easy to be able to talk to people whilst in the treatment room or salon.

a word of warning

Very occasionally you may come across a client you cannot get on with.

After over 21 years as a beauty therapist there have been only a handful of times when this has occurred, but it did happen, and the chances are it can and will happen to you at some point in your career. The strange thing is you never know why you find the relationship hard to form but the solution is simple. Book the client's next appointment with another therapist. You have heard the saying; 'you can't win them all'. Recognize that in the client's and salon's best interest introducing a different therapist will ensure a good relationship and a long-term client is almost guaranteed.

People tend to buy from someone they like and trust

Preparing to sell yourself

This chapter titled Selling Yourself is devoted to looking at the qualities and techniques a salesperson should adopt, plus some characteristics to aspire to.

But always remember:

- Learn from the experts.

- Copy sales techniques.

However, let your own personality shine through – always be yourself and be proud of it.

Qualities of a salesperson

Appearance – a trip down memory lane

Rewind your mind to your beauty college days. Now depending how far you have to go (in my case it was the white tights era as I call it in 1984, because as part of our standard uniform we always had to wear white tights) you will recall how on your first few days at beauty school you were almost 'brainwashed' about the importance of appearance. I have therefore prepared a quick checklist to re-inforce the key points. As you prepare to go on the salon floor, ask yourself the following questions:

- Is my uniform clean and pressed?

- Is my hair clean, neat and tidy?

- Are my shoes clean and comfortable?

- Is my make-up professionally applied and my skin looking healthy and well cared for?

- Are my nails well manicured?

- Is my jewellery kept to a minimum?

- Is my fragrance acceptable and discreet?

- And finally, is my leg tan well applied? – Not a white tight in sight!

Our industry focuses on helping people feel good and look good, so it is essential that we portray the right appearance in order to create a good first impression. Customers would feel uncomfortable if on their first visit to a slimming group the instructor was four stone overweight, this situation would not exactly inspire confidence. The same applies to us. We must show our clients that we care about our appearance and will therefore automatically care about theirs.

Getting your appearance right is essential. Think for a moment about the skin-care houses in department stores. Have you ever noticed how immaculate their sales assistants look no matter what time of day you see them? Initially, the only sales tool they have is their appearance. When customers walk into the store they have the choice of at least 20 people to approach for advice. Whilst it is true advertising, marketing and merchandising play a key part in the customers' choice, one deciding factor is the person behind the counter and the assistants know this. How would you feel if ten salons opened consecutively next to your salon? It is worrying enough if one opens half a mile away. Your appearance can initially make all the difference. Clients will look at you and ask themselves, 'do I want this person to be my beauty therapist?' Never underestimate the power of appearance.

The missing quality

Never in any appearance training are we told of the most important quality:

- the one that costs nothing yet pays dividends

- the one that is always there, yet we forget to use

- the one that creates the best first impression, the best lasting impression and

- the biggest impact …

> ### a smile … do not sell without it!

When you smile you feel good, furthermore, when you smile at someone it makes them feel good, this is a good start to building relationships. If you smile at someone they tend to smile back at you – go on try it.

When you smile you feel good.

When you smile I feel good.

When you smile I'll smile.

A passionate belief in what you retail

If you sell it use it. Having a strong and passionate belief in what you retail is essential. You must be convinced that you are offering your clients the best retail products. If you don't rate your products, then go out and find a range that you do. By selling something you do not believe in, you are breaking the golden rule of honesty in selling. Use your products at home and see the amazing results for yourself: during the sales presentation this genuine enthusiasm will shine through. There will always be certain products that are not suitable for you to use, so ask family or friends to try them and give you feedback. During the sales process your ability to recall positive testimonials about your products will not only increase your passion and belief but also your clients' likelihood to buy.

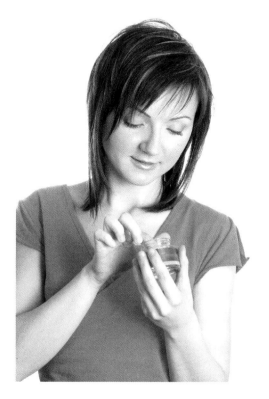

Use your products at home and see the amazing results for yourself

Your self-esteem and motivation levels will lift and you will have a firm positive grounding for selling.

Know your products – product knowledge versus passion

Although we deal with product knowledge in a later chapter, it is still an important quality for a salesperson. Product knowledge is an area of selling which has been the centre of much debate.

I have created many sales by using enthusiasm and passion for the products alone; I have also sold products with product knowledge alone. The truth is, you need a mixture of both; the degree to which each skill plays a role will vary from client to client.

A true professional salesperson makes it their business to know as much as possible about the products they sell. Later in this book you will find a whole chapter has been devoted to product knowledge including a 15-minute method to help you remember all you need to know about your products, their ingredients, benefits and the results they provide.

Listen, don't just hear

We hear things constantly, as our ears pick up noises, sounds and words. Hearing is often a subconscious sense. For example, when someone is talking you may be able to hear what they say but you do not necessarily have to listen, your mind can be elsewhere. With regard to selling, one of the greatest skills is to create an effective level of LISTENING.

characteristics that create a great listener include:

1 Notice not only what people say but also how they say it – 70 per cent of communication is non-verbal. Your clients will be constantly giving you clues about their feelings by their body language, tone of voice, even facial expressions.

2 Become an active listener – leaning slightly forward, making eye contact and giving a little nod as they are talking will encourage your clients and show you are listening.

3 Pause before replying – don't wait for your clients to take a breath then jump in to talk. A comfortable pause reassures your clients that you have been listening to what they have said.

4 Feed back what your clients have said – for example, 'let me make sure I understand your concerns' or 'what you are saying is…'. This has a twofold effect. Firstly, your clients will feel valued as they will realize you were actually listening. Secondly, your clients, listening to their own words repeated back to them, will tend to add more information about their concerns to add clarity. By effectively using your listening skills your clients will talk more.

The focus of attention is always on the person who is talking. It can help to think of it as a spotlight. Most of the time it should be shining on your clients, whenever you talk it shines on you; don't leave your clients in the dark for too long.

Begin now listening on this new level. The words you hear are only a small part of our listening skills. Implement the above four characteristics to enhance your listening skills and sales.

The ability to ask questions – excellent communication skills

The sales process requires effective communication through the asking of questions. Your aim is to ascertain your clients' needs through a series of questions in a relaxed conversational manner. We all have a natural and preferred manner of speech, within the sales process it has to be calm and client-focused without turning it into an interrogation.

By developing excellent questioning skills you will get your clients' attention and interest in their home-care routine and be able to guide the conversation towards the results you and your products can achieve.

 tip

Each and every time your clients visit you always begin by performing a mini consultation. Ask key questions regarding:

- The results of their last treatment.

- How the products they bought are performing.

- If you gave them any samples, ask if they enjoyed using them.

- Always ask if your clients have any specific concerns today.

High levels of confidence and self-esteem

How you feel about yourself and the level of belief in yourself will have a direct impact, not only on your ability to sell successfully, but also on the results you achieve. Highly successful salespeople are confident in their abilities to provide

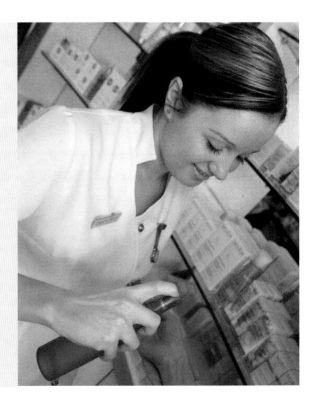

Applying basic courtesies will have a dramatic impact on results

the best solutions for their customers, concerns and that alone increases their self-esteem. We all have high levels of confidence in some areas of our life and the key is to learn to access our inner confidence and utilize it when selling. Confidence comes from taking small achievable steps towards our goal, making new choices, taking new challenges and aiming for excellence but not perfection. Aiming for perfection places an enormous amount of pressure on yourself and the chances are you will struggle to reach your goal. Excellence, however, is achievable, as it motivates and offers less chance of failure.

> If at first you don't succeed at selling, find out why and then change what you are doing. By focusing on the areas to improve, your confidence levels will remain intact.

Manners and respect

It is often said that it is the little things that make the biggest difference and applying small basic courtesies during the sales process will have a dramatic impact on the results you achieve.

> ### good old fashioned manners
> ### = MORE SALES

> ### having respect for your clients
> ### = MORE SALES

- Use the two magical words, please and thank you, make a habit of saying 'Thank you for your custom' to your clients.

- When you first meet your clients try saying 'It is a pleasure to meet you'.

- On their next visit, try saying 'It is lovely to see you again'.

- Respect your clients' views, never be critical or judgemental, listen to and value their opinions.

Create the right first impression. By using basic courtesy and manners the likelihood of clients buying from you will be increased.

 tip

- The sales process begins the moment your clients enter the salon, not when you place the products in front of them.

- The positive and warm way you welcome clients in to the salon will begin to create the right environment for selling.

Enjoy selling

To be good at a task it really helps if you enjoy doing it. Furthermore, the more you enjoy doing it the more likely you are to do it regularly. Enjoy selling, do not be too hard on yourself, get it all in perspective. Develop a good sense of humour and see the lighter side of selling. If you lose a sale just look for the next opportunity to gain a sale. Be optimistic and open minded, but above all have fun.

 tip

Please take this advice seriously, it is so important that you enjoy selling. Although I have immense passion, professionalism and focus when selling, I really do enjoy it as well. I would even hasten to add that I prefer selling to performing the treatments. I regularly set myself retail targets to achieve and constantly aim for higher retail sales. However, on the occasions I don't achieve my retail goals, I reward myself for the results I did achieve. I then try to think of new ways to reach my targets, but I always enjoy the process.

> **clients tend to buy from a therapist they like and trust**

✔ key reminders

- Dress for success. Your appearance speaks volumes.

- Believe in what you sell. If you sell it … use it.

- Successful selling requires a blend of product knowledge and enthusiasm.

- Become an active listener.

- Develop a relaxed conversational style when asking questions – avoid interrogating your clients.

- Believe in yourself and your abilities.

- Use good old fashioned manners.

- Remember to enjoy selling – have fun.

Exercises

1 a Read through the list of qualities of a salesperson. Place each item onto the chart on the next page according to your own proficiency.

   b Each item placed in the 'top performer' box are your strengths, focus on these during the sales process.

   c The qualities placed in the 'need to practise' box are ones that you know with a little more effort and focus will too become strengths.

   d Any item placed in the 'a lot to learn' box are your weaknesses and need to be developed and practised.

If you remember the 'wheel of selling', the sales process requires all of the parts to be successful. The same is true with qualities of a salesperson. Knowing your strengths and weaknesses gives you the winning edge to develop your sales potential.

TOP PERFORMER	
NEED TO PRACTISE	
A LOT TO LEARN	

qualities of a successful salesperson

- Professional appearance
- Thorough product knowledge – product features and benefits
- Excellent listener
- High levels of confidence and self-esteem
- Excellent manners and respect
- Enjoy selling
- Friendly
- Eager to please
- Good at building relationships with clients
- Very trustworthy and honest
- Solution orientated
- Maintain a positive attitude
- Excellent customer care skills
- Make every client feel important and special
- A passionate belief in what you retail
- Ability to ask questions

The door to success is labelled push!

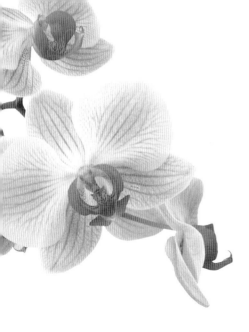

chapter four
relationship selling

Introduction

> ## people tend to buy from someone they like and trust

Relationship selling is probably the single most important factor in creating a successful and long-term sales career. Clients tend to buy and repeatedly buy from someone they like and trust. In other words people buy from someone they feel they have a good relationship with.

The old style of selling has gone: a quick sale, hit and run sale or, 'get the sale and go', belong in the past. Today we need repeat sales; a one-off sale will not keep your salon in business in the long term. The new salesperson has to give more, they have to be client focused and service orientated and make it easy and enjoyable for their clients to buy.

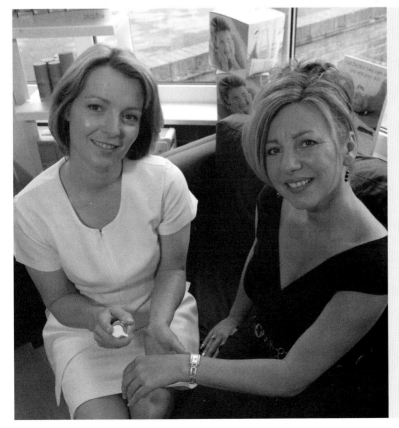

To keep your business going long term you need repeat sales

Within this chapter we will review:

- How vital it is to build a professional relationship with your clients

- The essential qualities that trust and honesty play in selling

- The new model of selling

- How to establish a rapport with your clients

- The importance of putting your clients at the heart of every sale

Building relationships

Building good relationships with your clients has to be your main focus during the sales process. Whilst many salespeople in other professions struggle to even get time with their customers, it is amazing how many of our clients will initially come to see us. Usually visiting to enjoy a treatment, it gives us a unique opportunity to build a great relationship with them. Focusing on relationships has to be the first step to achieving success in selling and that includes dream clients who walk through the salon door just to purchase products. The initial temptation is to close the sale, in other words, simply sell them the products they require. However, pause and try to establish some kind of relationship. These clients may walk into many salons and purchase products, your aim is to ensure that from now on the only salon they visits is yours and the only products they purchase are the ones you recommend.

Ideas to build this relationship could include:

- Offering a complementary skin consultation.

- Inviting them to enjoy a short treatment, which in turn could encourage them to book a complete treatment.

- Alternatively, you could include discount vouchers off their next product purchases or salon treatment.

Question

Think of a time when you bought something you later regretted. Maybe you felt pressured into buying, or felt you paid too much. How did you feel? Those negative and precautionary triggers are inside many potential clients, who can instantly replay many scenarios in their mind when they felt this way causing them to become suspicious when you try to sell. The key word here is YOU, you have to remove all their negative and limiting feelings and make their decision to buy easy and comfortable. Most sales that end in a 'No' do so because the clients view it as a risk. It is not the lowest price clients look for but rather the lowest risk. You have to lower your clients' perception of risk by building a good relationship. Therefore, how your clients see and feel about you is vital.

Your relationship with your clients is the heart of the sales process; it is the catalyst that brings everything else together.

> As a therapist you should make it both easy and enjoyable for your clients to buy.

Relationship building skills

As I have previously discussed, the relationship between clients and their therapist is so crucial you have to get it right from the start.

The two skills which can have the biggest impact are establishing a rapport with you clients and being trustworthy and honest.

Establishing rapport

People tend to buy from someone they like. A dictionary definition of rapport is:

> ## a harmonious understanding within a relationship

Within the selling context we need to ensure our communications are effective and that as salespeople we can adapt to individual clients. People like people who are similar to themselves and therefore having a flexible personality, whilst remaining true to your values, is a great skill. As therapists we find that we already have the ability to gain rapport with many different kinds of people. Building relationships is a core skill within selling and I believe beauty therapists have a head start over most professions in this area.

Trust and honesty

> **people tend to buy from someone they trust**

To be trusted you must be trustworthy. During my years as a beauty therapist I have developed a reputation for honesty. I never recommended treatments or sold products if I did not believe they would benefit my clients. I have even been known to recommend another salon's treatment or product range if I felt they would offer a better solution to my clients' concerns. One of the greatest compliments I received from a client was 'The honest advice Ruth gives makes a refreshing change, she has my best interests at heart not how much money she can make from me.'

Always give honest advice, let your clients feel the trust and this alone will ensure long-term relationships with them. It pays to be honest; it is a vital ingredient of every single sales transaction.

At the heart of every sale are your clients, their needs, their views and their feelings:

- focus on your clients
- concentrate on the relationship
- put the clients' needs first, and
- watch the sales follow.

real life example

keep caring and eventually you will sell

I can recall one particular client who would never buy any products that I recommended. On her first visit to the salon she made it clear that she enjoyed using her existing products and had no desire to change or purchase any more products.

Every visit I would perform a mini skin consultation, ask what she would like to achieve from the treatment and if she had any particular concerns. Each time the same responses were given – 'I just want to relax today and no, I have no concerns'. If during the consultation I pointed out a concern regarding her skin, she would expect the treatment to help it. This went on for a few months.

Then I decided to change my approach. I had noticed my client's skin was quite dehydrated and dull, so instead of recommending my products, I asked her to bring in all her home-care range to the salon on her next visit. I mentioned that although she was happy with her existing range she may not be using them correctly. I focused on helping my client, on building a trustworthy relationship. Step by step, I showed her how to correctly cleanse, tone and hydrate her skin using her products, in other words, I educated her. My client thanked me and commented that no one had ever shown her how to do this before. I still refrained from selling to her, instead I gave her some samples of products that would not only benefit her skin but also work well with her existing products.

On her next visit … nothing … no sales! 'Oh well, I thought, 'at least I tried.'

However, on the following visit she asked me to recommend a night cream as she had just run out. Her reason for buying from me was simple. I had taken the time to help her; I had demonstrated that I cared about her skin and her, so in my client's opinion I deserved her business.

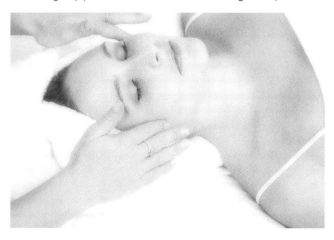

Giving honest advice will build the trust of your client

Work customer care and selling together

The link between customer care and selling is very strong. The two should never be isolated in our goal to build long-term sales.

> ## if you desire to sell well you must serve well

I said in Chapter 1 that there is no magic formula to selling, but if there is a magic ingredient when you sell, it must be the absolute determination to give excellent customer care. From the moment your clients enter the salon to the moment they leave, they must be offered a five-star treatment and first-class service.

There are always ways to improve your customer care in the salon. The way you greet or welcome your clients, the care you offer in the treatment room right through to the clients, leaving the salon, all affect their perception of you and their overall salon experience. Generally look at ways to improve your clients' salon experience and the care they receive whilst in your salon.

✔ key reminders

- People tend to buy from someone they like and trust.
- Focusing on relationship selling will put you in the top 10 per cent of salespeople.
- People like people who are similar to themselves.
- Honesty has to be in every sales process.

Exercises

Techniques for building rapport and relationships

Write down the eight key techniques that will help you establish rapport with your clients. To help you find them, think what you do when you first meet people. What would you say? How would you treat new clients?

1

2

3

4

5

6

7

8

A smile … don't sell
without it

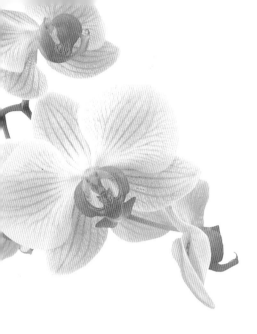

chapter five
the consultation

Introduction

I use the heading 'Consultation' as it is one we are so familiar with. We understand it to be a process of obtaining information from our clients through a series of questions. The aim of this stage is to uncover your clients' needs and concerns, wants or desires, in other words this stage is all about RESEARCH. The consultation is a time when you focus on asking a series of key questions to fully understand your clients' situations before you can make recommendations and present your solutions. Verbal communication is a two-way process; as well as asking questions you have to listen to your clients' responses.

you will learn

Within this chapter we will review:

- How to perform a professional consultation

- The application of open and closed questions

- The three roles for successful selling

always ask – never assume

Asking questions and listening to the response

Never assume you know what your clients want or need; by taking this approach apart from losing sales you are undervaluing your clients by not letting their views matter. Imagine visiting your doctor and explaining your ailment, how would you feel if no questions were asked, a short diagnosis made and a prescription quickly written? Apart from feeling worried that no investigating questions were asked or the area examined, you would leave with no confidence in the diagnosis and little faith in the prescription. Taking the time to ask questions and listen to your clients' responses is vital whether you are performing a complete skin consultation or simply advising on a product.

The importance of asking questions is best illustrated during an electrolysis consultation. In order for clients to qualify for treatment and to assess the success of the treatment the cause of hair growth must be ascertained. After over 21 years of performing electrolysis consultations I never assume I know the cause. I ask relevant questions, listen to the responses, feed the important points back to my clients for clarification, and ask more questions until I uncover the cause. Experience has taught me that there are too many causes of hair growth to jump to conclusions. Now compare this to the selling situation, where similarly you need to know everything in order to recommend the correct products.

> Keep a deep interest in solving your clients' concerns; knowing what is important to them is only achievable through questioning.

The three roles for successful selling

Follow the detective, doctor, therapist (DDT) technique when selling and not only will you solve all your clients' concerns, and increase your level of sales in an efficient and professional manner, but you will be putting your clients at the heart of the sales process. Whilst we look at the importance of each role individually they are not meant to be in any particular order. In many situations I have begun with the 'doctor' role as I felt it vital to look at the skin condition first. What is important is that the concept of each role plays a part during the sales process.

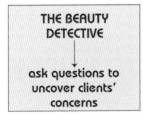

THE BEAUTY DETECTIVE

ask questions to uncover clients' concerns

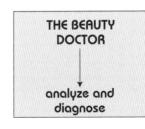

THE BEAUTY DOCTOR

analyze and diagnose

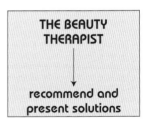

THE BEAUTY THERAPIST

recommend and present solutions

utilize each role during the sales process

Strange as it may sound, if you imagine these three character roles and absorb yourself into the principles of each of them (you should have no problems with one of them) you will refrain from rushing to the recommending stage of selling as so many of us do. Instead you will take a little time to gather information through a series of questions, then make a diagnosis, give advice and demonstrate your product. During my sales training programme I use props to reinforce these roles. For example, a policeman's helmet for the detective role. This part of the training provokes so much fun that the principle of asking key questions when selling is never forgotten.

 tip

Most therapists' sales are low because they rush to the recommending stage of selling.

Your first role – be a beauty detective

You are aiming to solve your clients' concerns so think of yourself as a detective. The only way to solve their problems is to ask lots of relevant questions and keep asking until you fully understand the situation. Each client is different and therefore each series of questions you ask will vary from client to client. It is therefore imperative to develop sets of questions for each area you sell in. For example, skin care, body care, nail care. The quality of your ques-

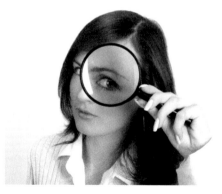

As a beauty detective you must keep asking your client relevant questions

tions will affect the conversation and client involvement, so use a mixture of encouraging and involvement questions. These type of questions involve the client and cause them to participate, as well as inspiring them to communicate, e.g. 'It is great you enjoy using products as home. What routine do you have and how much time do you devote to it?'

OPEN QUESTIONS – This type of question always begins with why, what, who, when, where or how. Open questions 'open' the conversation and require a conversational style answer. An example would be: 'What skin-care products are you currently using?' or 'What are your key concerns regarding your skin?'

CLOSED QUESTIONS – This type of question will receive a yes or a no or a one-word answer as the response. Closed questions can limit your research. However, they are great to use for clarification. An example would be: 'Do you currently use a night treatment cream?' or 'Do you prefer a wash-off cleanser or cleansing milk?' or 'So today you are looking for a high performance eye cream to help diminish the fine lines and wrinkles?'

When you ask a question link your next question to your client's response.

THERAPIST: 'What kind of cleansing routine or product are you using at the moment?'

CLIENT: 'I am using a gel that I wash off.'

THERAPIST: 'Do you prefer using water when cleansing?'

CLIENT: 'Oh yes, I can't be bothered using cotton wool.'

To gain more information a great question would be:

THERAPIST: 'How do you mean exactly?'

CLIENT: 'Well it just takes too long and I don't feel clean afterwards'.

How many times have we heard that?

After asking a few questions it is important to feed back to your client what has been said; this feedback technique has many advantages:

1 It helps gain clarification on the information you have received.

2 When the client hears her own words back she may add more information.

3 It shows the client you have been actively listening.

4 It keeps the conversation focused on the subject.

An example of a feedback question would be:

THERAPIST: 'So you do cleanse your skin twice a day with a wash-off gel cleanser which gives you a really clean feeling afterwards which is important to you?'

CLIENT: 'Yes, but I only cleanse at night, in the morning I just wash my face in the shower.'

In this example the feedback question clarified the information but the client added she only cleanses once a day so immediately our questions have uncovered another valuable clue.

Another tip, if you keep asking feedback questions the chances are they will end in a 'yes', this helps put the client in a positive frame of mind and gets her used to saying yes – really useful when closing the sale!

Listening as a beauty detective

Actively listening to your clients' responses is the hallmark of a great salesperson. Your clients will tell you all you need to know by what they say, by how they say it and by their body language. All you have to do is listen and listen well to collect all the facts and information. The clues are there.

> **listen and you will hear**

The detective role uncovers concerns or your clients' needs that require solving, so your questions have to be information seeking. Take notes during this stage as later you will need to match your clients' needs with the benefits of your products and you don't want to forget any.

Once you have uncovered your clients' concerns it is time to swap hats and become a beauty doctor.

real life example

the questions that were never asked

I chose to emphasize the importance of asking questions during professional selling because it is the one area that:

- is usually performed quickly or else forgotten

- will totally involve your clients and make them feel important

- will give you most of the information you need to successfully sell.

Over the many years I have observed therapists selling, I am totally amazed by the lack of questions clients are asked. For example:

A client enters the salon reception and asks if they can speak to a beauty therapist for advice.

CLIENT: 'I find that no matter what cleanser I use I still keep getting small blemishes on my skin, even some underneath it.'

THERAPIST: 'Which cleansers have you tried?'

CLIENT: 'Most on the market! I have had enough of spending money on products that do not work.'

THERAPIST: 'Well try this one [therapist removes a product from the shelf] this will work.'

Now this is not an extreme example – this is a case history and I have seen it in action many times. Let's now replay this scenario and add some simple basic questioning.

CLIENT: 'I find that no matter what cleanser I use I still keep getting small blemishes on my skin, even some underneath it.'

THERAPIST: 'Which cleaners have you tried, for example, wash-off cleansers or cleansing milk?'

CLIENT: 'Most on the market! I have tried all types of cleansing products; none of them have made any difference.'

THERAPIST: 'Please could you tell me some of the ones you have tried?'

CLIENT: 'Well I have tried brand x, brand y, brand z.'

(From the client's response it is clear that she has tried quality products, ones that would normally give a good result.)

THERAPIST: 'Those products are premium quality; they should have worked. May I ask you a few more questions regarding your home-care routine?'

CLIENT: 'Yes, certainly.'

THERAPIST: 'Apart from cleansing what else do you do to your skin?'

CLIENT: 'I exfoliate twice a week, I apply a day cream, and a night cream and apply treatment masks weekly.'

real life example continued

(From the client's response it is clear that there must be another reason her skin is continually suffering from small blemishes.)

THERAPIST: 'May I ask if you regularly wear make-up?'

CLIENT: 'Every day! I never go anywhere without my make-up on.'

THERAPIST: 'Could you please tell me which make up you use?'

CLIENT: 'I use brand x I have been using it for years.'

AHA! Now we have the real reason for the client's skin concern. The foundation she is using is one that stays on the skin and has to be removed with the aid of an oil-based remover prior to skin cleansing.

Simply by asking six straightforward questions to the client we have ascertained the cause of the problem and can recommend a suitable product for the client to purchase.

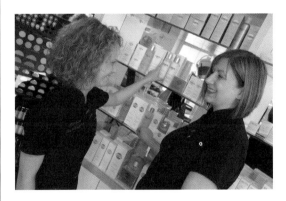

Following the detective, doctor, therapist technique puts your client at the heart of the selling process

Now it's time to examine and analyze

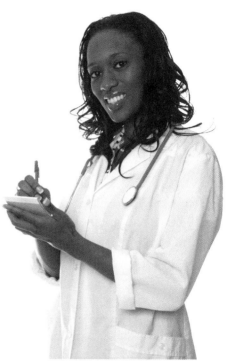

Your second role – be a beauty doctor

Now it is time to examine and analyze. You will have gathered lots of relevant information through your detective work and now it is time to start piecing it together by looking at the concern and giving your professional diagnosis. If your clients have just enjoyed a treatment you would have had ample time and opportunity to look at their skin. When clients just book for a consultation, you start your observations immediately.

A tip which I find very powerful during this stage is to always pay your clients a compliment, but it must be a genuine one or they will see straight through it. Over the years, clients have approached me for advice with concerns such as acne or eczema and in each case their self-esteem can be very low and they can be feeling very negative about their appearance. Therefore I find something positive and pay them a compliment, which in turn makes them focus on a positive and they feel better about themselves. It may be their beautiful long lashes or their lovely thick long hair, both of which I would love, so the compliment is genuine and it comes across as such. As long as compliments are genuine and honest they will help to build the relationship with your clients.

At this point of the sales process you are identifying what the concerns are by using your knowledge and experience. Always talk to your clients during the skin and body analysis part, give positive feedback and ask more questions to clarify and gain more information.

Now you have gathered all your information, analyzed and diagnosed, it is time to move on to the next role. This is the role we know and love best – the beauty therapist.

Your third role – be yourself – the beauty therapist

This part of the sales process is devoted to prescribing, presenting and demonstrating products. Your aim is to successfully link your product benefits to your clients' needs to solve their problems and deliver the required results. The next chapter is totally devoted to presenting and demonstrating effectively to achieve high level of sales.

Tips and techniques for effective consultations

1 FOCUS on the REASONS your clients visit you. The main part of the conversation has to be result focused.

2 Ask questions that reveal which products clients are using now and ones they have used in the past. Not only will this information give you a clear picture of their home-care routine and the type and texture of products they like, but it will also tell you how much money they are used to spending on products.

3 Ask questions to uncover your clients' desires. Discover what they really want to achieve from their home-care programme. During a recent skin-care consultation a client expressed her concern about her dry skin. It was only

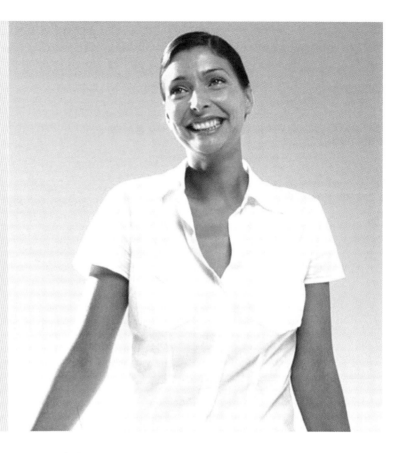

Be yourself – the
beauty therapist

after I had recommended the products and explained how her skin would
benefit in just a short period of time, that she then explained the one thing
she would love is to get rid of these red marks on her cheeks. The thread
veins on her cheeks were the one thing she really wanted to improve. After a
short explanation, I re-booked my client for a thread vein removal
consultation and treatment.

4 Be realistic and honest about what your products will do. In the above
   example my client initially thought that the products she purchased would
   help fade her red marks. I was honest and explained they could only be
   removed by a salon treatment. Do not set the stage for failure.

if you lie your sales will eventually die

5 Throughout a consultation try and guide as opposed to control the conversation. In my life coaching training if the conversation goes off track, we guide our clients by bringing them back to the issues being discussed. You are helping your clients to achieve results, be professional and focus on helping them understand how well your products will work. Your clients' feelings are an essential part of the sales process, treat them with respect.

6 Never knock any products your clients may be using now: effectively you are undermining their previous buying decisions and by doing so you will erect an enormous barrier against successful selling. We have all made purchasing mistakes in the past and the last thing we need is for someone to remind us of them, or tell us that we were wrong to buy them.

7 When analyzing or diagnosing, give your clients a hand-held mirror to involve them and show them your observations. It portrays a caring approach and a professional interest on your part. Another tip: try not to lay clients flat on the couch; as more of a sitting-up position works better.

8 Always begin your conversation with no products, concentrate on building the relationship and trust by asking key questions to identify needs. Compare the following two scenarios.

9 Don't always look for clients' needs. These days customers are more knowledgeable regarding skin-care. Many clients are already following a skin-care programme.

You decide to introduce a new skin-care range into your salon and you invite two representatives into your salon from their respective companies:

representative 1 – from skin-care company A
The representative arrives at your salon loaded down with products, cases, laptop and leaflets. They get the pleasantries over with and then go into automatic selling – the presentation they deliver to ALL salon owners. They tell us how good their products are, how so many salons do so well with them, perform a standard demonstration then sit back and expect us to say 'Great I'll take the lot'. If we don't, they then say how wrong we would be if we don't stock their products. By the way, this is not an extreme example, I have experienced this many times.

representative 2 – from skin-care company B

The representative walks into your salon with no products (yes we know they are in the boot of their car), instead a file with pre-prepared questions to ask you. They initiate a good conversation to establish rapport and pay you or your salon a genuine compliment. They then say 'Ruth, I believe our products will help your business tremendously, but first may I ask you a few questions before I show and explain them to you?' They ask about existing treatments we offer, products we retail and what we want to achieve through stocking a new skin-care range. From our responses they ask more questions taking a deep interest in our current situation. Then, and only then, will the representative start linking the benefits of their products to the salon needs and how the range will deliver the results we require. The presentation is then tailored to our requirements, initially demonstrating the product areas we have shown an interest in.

question

Now ask yourself which company would you like to do business with?

Clients already know they need the products; your role is to find out what they require. What is their existing skin-care range or routine lacking? The need has already been established, you have to ask questions to identify and meet their new requirements.

10 During the consultation start creating desire or planting the seeds for your products. Use your concert selling points (see Chapter 7, Product Knowledge) to initiate desire and interest.

11 Keep your questions simple and easy to answer during the consultation. Your clients need to feel comfortable, so avoid technical jargon which will only confuse them and begin to alienate them from the conversation.

12 Don't interrogate your clients. Keep the conversation relaxed and flowing, encourage clients' involvement and don't forget to keep smiling.

13 Be professional. Be a consultant. Focus on helping people and delivering results. Your clients have the opportunity to visit shops or stores yet have chosen to come to you for advice. They expect a professional, caring approach so make sure you offer it.

real life example

build the relationship first

I recently received a telephone call from a client requesting a consultation. She had just returned from her holiday and had incredibly dry skin all over her body. She wished to purchase some products. Now my initial reaction was to have the products already in the room when she arrived. After all there was only going to be a few options: a body exfoliator, body oil and a treatment cream. Instead, I asked key questions and involved the client in the diagnosis and then I brought in the products. I established rapport, built trust, care and interest into the relationship first.

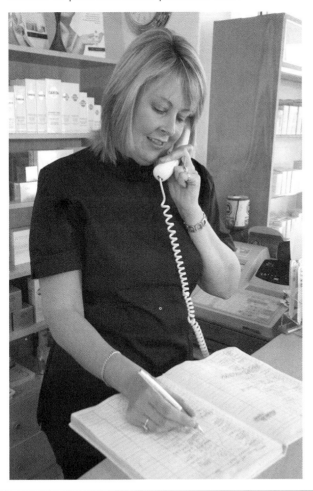

Involving the client in the diagnostic process establishes a rapport and builds trust

14 Avoid waiting until the end of the treatment before you begin talking about retail sales. Depending on the situation (either a new or existing client) try following the advice below.

    a Prior to the treatment sit down with your clients and discuss their concerns.

    b Begin planting the seed for retail sales. Discuss how you can tailor the treatment to their personal requirements by using your advanced skin-care range.

    c Now mention that you have an amazing product or products that will solve their concerns and give remarkable results. Then ask 'Would you like me to show you the products at the end of your treatment?', or 'I would like to introduce you to a new, effective and result-orientated home-care routine. Will that be convenient at the end of your treatment?'

I have been using this technique for the past 20 years and to date I have never had a client say no. Clients are therefore giving you permission to begin the sales process.

Below are sample questions for a skin consultation. However, these are just the beginning to steer you in the right direction. Try to add more questions yourself.

1 What are your key concerns?

2 What skin type do you feel you have?

3 What do you like about your skin?

4 What areas are you most concerned about?

5 What changes would you like to achieve?

6 In what areas do you want to see the biggest improvement?

7 How would you describe your skin?

8 How does your skin feel first thing in the morning?

9 What skin-care products are you currently using?

10 Have you ever tried the products we retail?

11 How effective do you find your current skin-care products?

12 What do you like about your current skin-care products?

13 Do you feel your existing products are delivering results?

14 Do you regularly use a foundation?

15 What kind of cleansing product do you use?

16 Does your skin ever feel taut, dry, greasy or sensitive?

17 How are you currently moisturising your skin?

18 Do you apply a night treatment product?

19 What specialized products do you apply to your eyes, lips and neck?

20 How often do you exfoliate your skin?

21 Do you apply face masks?

22 Do you suffer from any allergies?

23 Lifestyle has a major impact on our skin. Do you spend time in air
   conditioning or central heating or a lot of time outdoors?

✔ key reminders

- Uncover your clients' needs through asking key questions – think research.

- Never assume you know what your clients want.

- Remember the three key roles – detective, doctor, therapist. An effective consultation and a sales process requires all three to be successful.

Exercises

1 From the list of sample questions for a skin consultation, choose ten and
   copy them onto a separate sheet.

2 Immediately use these questions in your next skin consultation.

3 Evaluate the results and add two more questions from the list or add your own.

4 Keep repeating steps one to three until you have developed your own unique set of questions.

If you **tell** me ... I will forget, If you **show** me ... I may remember, If you **involve** me ... I will buy

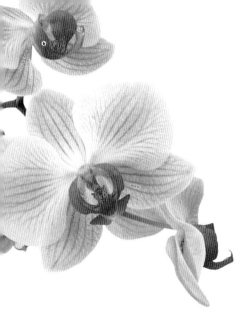

chapter six

product demonstration and presentation

Introduction

Salon products and services are constantly being improved and updated. In order to prosper in a competitive marketplace, salon professionals must be able to sell their products to both new and existing clients. Beauty therapists need to be able to provide solutions to their clients' concerns by selling their products through effective product demonstrations.

We are always reminded that customer care is not a spectator sport and neither is selling. The more you involve your customers when presenting and demonstrating the products the more you will increase their desire to purchase them and the higher your retail sales will be.

you will learn

Within this chapter we will review:

- How to correctly match the clients' needs and concerns with product features and benefits

- How to select the most appropriate time to inform your clients about home-care products

- How to use all five senses during the product demonstration

- How to give accurate and sufficient information to enable your clients to make buying decisions

- How to provide enough time for clients' questions and how to respond effectively to them

- How to understand the difference between product features and benefits

- How to educate clients to use their products correctly

- How to incorporate professional knowledge into your presentation

Now it is personal. Each presentation has to be personalized to your clients. Whilst you may follow basic guidelines, ensure each presentation is tailored to individual clients.

Demonstration and presentation

During the consultation you will have uncovered your clients' needs, now match these needs with the benefits of your products.

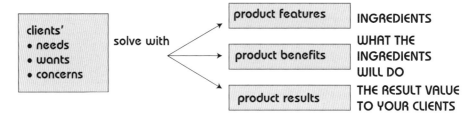

For example:

Your client's concern is a sensitive and reactive skin.

Product features – Lavender and cotton vegetable cells.

Product benefit – Immediately reduces inflammation and redness, whilst leaving a protective film on the skin.

Product result – Your skin will instantly look and feel calmer and soothed. It will regain its softness and the hydration levels of a normal healthy skin. After one week of use the results will be amazing – a healthy radiant skin.

think results! results! results!

Every time you recommend a product to your clients imagine them saying 'so what?', this is a very powerful technique which rapidly ensures you add on what the product will do for them and what the result will be.

During the presentation always ask yourself 'Am I achieving the desired outcome my clients want?' If during the consultation you uncovered that your clients' main concern is, for instance, fine lines around the eye area, then ensure your product presentation focuses initially on this need. Begin your demonstration by showing your clients the home-care products that will improve their concerns. This approach will make your clients more likely to buy.

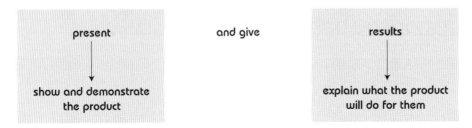

Your aim is for clients to clearly understand that by using a particular product their concerns will be met and their problems solved.

Product features and benefits

In Chapter 7, Product Knowledge, we shall discuss product features and benefits in greater detail. It is however important to understand the main difference between the two.

> A feature is a characteristic of the product, e.g. an ingredient.
>
> A benefit is what that feature will do for your clients and the results it will give.

For example, this day cream contains an SPF 15 (FEATURE) to help protect your skin from the sun's harmful rays (BENEFIT) which in turn can help prevent premature skin ageing (RESULT).

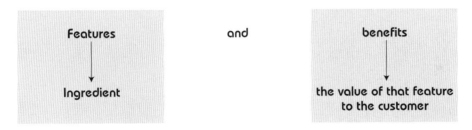

Clients do not buy features, they buy benefits. Whilst a knowledge of product features has a necessary role to play during the sales process (see Chapter 7) it is the product benefits that will ultimately lead to a sale.

> In reality, clients do not buy products; they buy the benefit of what the products will do for them.
>
> People buy solutions!

real life example

the rule of three

During many of the sales presentations I have observed, the area of selling the benefits is one that could be greatly improved by remembering 'the rule of three'. When explaining the product benefits to your clients only talk about three. Your clients will find it easy to remember three points regarding a product; they will clearly understand all the information and be able to see how they will benefit from using it.

Many therapists I have observed recall every single benefit imaginable. If you take this approach, for example by discussing six, seven or even more points, your clients can become over-loaded with information. Think of it this way, every time you mention a new benefit you will be simply diluting the previous information you have said and your clients will begin to switch off. Keep the points to a minimum, they will have a greater impact, are more likely to be remembered and will lead to a quicker buying decision. To select your three benefits simply choose the ones which match the clients' concerns.

Understand the difference between product features and benefits

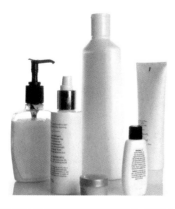

Product demonstration

Test drive your products

Interaction is the key word during a demonstration. You should aim for your clients to touch and apply each and every product.

If you were going to buy a new car the chances are you would test drive it first. By letting your clients test drive the products not only will they focus more on what you are doing and feel the benefits, but by using the products it creates ownership of them.

Handle with care

The way you handle your products will send a powerful message to your clients; treat your products with care.

- Hold the products as if they are an expensive piece of china.

- Decant products by using a small clean spatula.

- Ensure all your products are dust free and clean inside the lid and rim where the product can get trapped.

- Try not to use salon-size products for the demonstration for two reasons. Firstly, they are never packaged as nicely as retail products and can look bland. Secondly, they tend to be at least three times larger and the client may be disappointed when they see their size of product.

- Using a clean well-stocked tester stand to demonstrate from is very effective, but it is not always possible to have one in each treatment room. Try using a nice tray or product holder to take the products into the treatment room as opposed to carrying (or should I say balancing) them in your arms and placing them on the couch. A good idea is to place a product brochure and your clients' skin-care guide on the holder (what about a small vase of flowers?). Presentation is the key, so really focus on every little detail.

Correct home-care guidance

When explaining to your clients HOW to use the recommended products, follow these simple guidelines.

- Show your clients how much of the product to use. I refer to salon ranges as premium skin-care lines. I always explain to clients that my products are of an exceptional quality and therefore they only need to use a small amount.

- Demonstrate how to break down the product, by this I mean how to gently rub or warm up the product between the finger tips.

 tip

> Many clients will have never been shown how to apply products correctly. Your role is to show them the correct way to use their products through a professional demonstration. In my experience clients are almost afraid to ask the correct way to cleanse or apply creams. In all my years of selling I have never been stopped by a client whilst I have been demonstrating how to use products. All clients love to either learn the basics or be reassured they are using their products correctly.

- Show clients where to put the product, for example, where exactly to apply an eye cream, or when applying creams to include the neck and décolleté.

- Ensure clients are aware of how often to use the product. Is it twice a day? If prescribing a mask is it once or twice a week?

To recap:

1   Select the correct product.

2   Show the correct amount.

3   Demonstrate how to warm the product.

4   Show where to apply the product.

5   Explain how often to use the product.

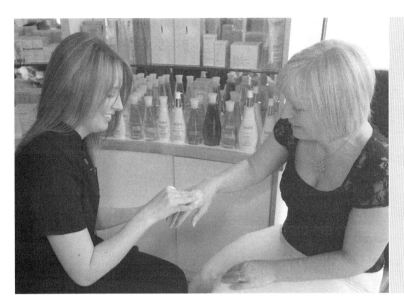

Demonstrate to your clients the correct way to use the products

Use all five senses when demonstating

Hearing

As you demonstrate and present your products what you are saying and how you are saying it is having a tremendous impact on your clients' buying decision. Your clients should be hearing positive and result-orientated words and phrases such as:

'This product is a true delight to use.'
'This is our best selling face mask.'
'Just feel how rapidly the cream absorbs into your skin.'
'There has never been anything quite like this product.'
'This is one of my personal favourites.'
'Isn't the texture amazing?'

Keep involving the client through asking questions such as:

'How does that texture feel?' or
'Do you like the aroma of the product?'

Touch

Letting clients touch and feel the products will create an inner feeling of owner-ship. To many clients how the product feels or works on their skin is their prime concern. By ensuring your clients try the products you will erase many fears and future objections will be overcome. For example, as your clients are applying their product back up their actions with a positive reinforcement.

'This product has an amazing affinity with the skin'

or

'What sets our products apart is their exceptional texture, just feel the quality of it.'

Smell

Isn't it amazing: if you tell someone a product has no aroma they will still smell it. Watch the next time you see someone test a product (including yourself), one of the first actions they do is to smell it. Do not underestimate the power of this sense, as aroma creates inner feelings of acceptance of the product. Apart from lemon, I personally don't like fruity aromas in products, no particular reason I just don't like them, I prefer floral aromas. Sense of smell, likes and dislikes is a very personal thing and can be difficult to detect. It may be a good idea to intro-duce a sample product during the consultation stage to almost check your clients like the aroma of your chosen product range. One thing is for sure, if clients don't like the aroma of the product they are unlikely to buy it.

Sight

Seeing is believing. An excellent visual presentation is one of the keys to suc-cessful selling. Trying to sell without the product in front of your clients can be done, indeed I have sold many products through passionate verbal communica-tion alone, but these sales tend to be to long-established clients where the trust bond is very strong. It is much easier to sell when there is a visual impact within the sales process.

Common sense

Be adaptable with your presentation, no two should be identical. Read your clients' body language; are there any buying signals or have they completely lost interest? Are they asking questions about the products, or are they completely silent?

Tell – show – tell

Here is a technique which is useful to remember when demonstrating products.

It is so simple yet so effective. With each product:

Tell   –   explain what product you are going to demonstrate and why.

Show   –   demonstrate the product and proceed to link the benefits of the product to your clients' concerns.

Tell   –   recap, clarify and summarize what you have just done to reinforce the results that will be gained from using the product.

An example would be:

TELL – 'I have selected this neck cream as it will help improve the crepe skin on the neck and décolleté area which you are concerned with.'

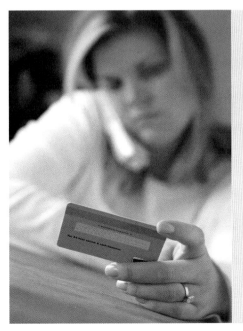

Shopping channels achieve amazing beauty product sales just through the power of words

SHOW – 'I will just take a few moments to show you how to correctly apply the product to achieve the best results.' [Proceed with demonstration.]'

TELL – 'As you can see the product absorbs beautifully into the skin, you can feel and see the difference immediately due to the light-reflecting molecules. After only a few days your skin's texture will have dramatically improved due to the constant drip feed provided by the liposomes in the product.'

Selling the benefits

Over recent years teleshopping has become a major retailer of beauty products to the general public. Views on whether this is right or wrong is not the issue here but what is amazing is the volume of products they retail by selling the product benefits and results. It is really worth watching these programmes just to get fresh ideas on selling. The presenter takes every feature and then whole-heartedly turns it into a benefit and then focuses on the amazing results the products will give.

The presenters only have this one technique at their disposal. You can't touch, feel or smell the products, yet through the power of result selling amazing sales levels are achieved. They have to sustain interest through the words they use, so with this in mind let's look at words that can help increase your clients' desire to buy.

Words that sell

Below is a selection of phrases and words that will help you sell. They can be used during any part of the sales process and when used correctly can be very powerful.

'The results of this product are impressive.'
'This product really works.'
'It is the ultimate product.'
'A sensational feeling.'
'It is exquisite.'
'Just feel the amazing quality of this product.'

'These products are for those who appreciate quality.'
'This cream is a break-through formula that delivers results.'
'A unique formula.'
'Quality is what sets our products apart from other ranges on the market.'
'These products can be counted on to deliver results.'
'This product is a pure delight to use.'
'This cream will provide spectacular results.'

Extra tips and techniques for product demonstrations

- When showing your clients a product give it to them to hold, by doing so you are creating an element of ownership.

- If your clients have just had a treatment and you used some of the products that you are now presenting to them, comment on how great their skin looked and felt when you applied the products, adding how they really suited their skin.

 tip

- Always give clients a choice, instead of showing just one product show two or three.
- It is easy to say no to one but not as easy to two or three.

- If you want to sell three products present six to your clients and then focus the presentation on the three products as their key purchases.

- Show the complete picture. Where you are recommending a complete home-care programme explain to your clients that you will show them all the products they will eventually need. However, when you present them focus more on the essentials that they should purchase today.

- Create pictures in your clients' mind. When selling the results use descriptive words that will create a picture in your clients' imagination. This visualization technique will increase your clients' desire to buy by almost seeing the results in advance. For example, you might say how after three weeks of using this eye cream it will minimize fine lines and wrinkles and signs of fatigue, or after just one application of this mask your skin will glow and look so radiant. Create a picture of how your clients' skin will look and feel after using this product.

- Your clients may already be following an effective skin-care routine and have no major concerns. In this example refrain from trying to recommend a complete new range. Remember, our aim is to keep your customers as treatment clients. Within all our product ranges we have what I refer to as unique products. Ones that many other ranges do not have. Within one of the ranges we retail are essential oils and these products can be added to any existing skin-care routine. One of the immediate benefits of using these products is amazing skin radiance. With the above scenario I would simply ask my clients if they would like to see a product that will give their skin radiance and a really healthy appearance. Undoubtedly your clients will say yes. You will have gained a sale and introduced your clients to your products without undermining their existing range. Consequently as their other products run out your clients will turn to you for advice and future purchases.

The 'beautiful selling' prescription guide

The 'beautiful selling' prescription guide is what will set you apart from other sales people in our profession. This sales tool is powerful, effective and will improve your sales performance as soon as you start using it.

Over the next few pages I have illustrated a sample and once tailored to your salon and products print out this unique guide and implement immediately.

By providing your clients with a personal prescription guide you will:

- dramatically increase your sales

- have an excellent tool to use during your presentation to link benefits to clients' concerns

- show your clients you really care and have taken the time to prescribe and develop their personalized home-care programme (see pages 79–82).

Page 1 – front cover

Personalize – add client's name and your salon details

Page 2

product:	key ingredients:	benefits/results:
Write down product name and two options to give clients a choice	Write down an easy to understand (and pronounce) ingredient e.g. floral waters. By listing one or two ingredients you are showing your knowledge and professionalism.	Link at least two benefits of the product to the clients' concerns Show you are solving their problems by selling the result.

Page 3

How to use your products:

Although you would have demonstrated how to use your products this page acts as a back-up for your clients at home. It shows you are a true professional and you have again taken the time to go that extra mile. Most clients forget how and when to use their products, this page will remind them and ensure they get the results they desire.

Page 4

Your personal guide to purchasing your products:

After your presentation many clients will ask which products to take first. This section allows you to list in order of priority to help clients make their decision.

Avoid: 1 Cleanser
2 Toner
3 Day cream

Clients will probably just purchase 1 and 2 – the cleanser and the toner

Instead: 1 Cleanser, Toner, Day cream, Exfoliater
2 Night cream, Eye mask
3 Neck gel, Face mask, etc.

In this example clients are more likely to purchase the cleanser, toner, day cream and exfoliater.

Recommended salon treatments

This space is for you to advise on future treatments for your clients and encourages them to book further appointments.

Next skin analysis

Here you can write a date when your client's next skin analysis should be performed – remember, you are aiming for a long-term relationship – you want and need your clients to revisit the salon.

> this is again focusing on a long-term relationship with your clients

✔ key reminders

- Match your clients' needs to the product benefits.
- Involve your clients in the presentation.
- Think results, results, results.
- Use all five senses during your presentation.
- Use words that sell.
- Always give your clients a choice.

Exercises

Using the sample of the *Beautiful Selling Prescription Guide*, adapt it to your salon and product ranges. Design a proof, then have it printed and implement it immediately. Then watch the sales follow.

welcome to the world of

(name of your skin-care range here)

....

your personal prescription guide

add photo	add photo	add photo

add salon name here

add salon address and telephone number here

home-care product recommendation

to clean your skin – a healthy skin begins with effective cleansing

product:	key ingredients:	benefits:	results:

to exfoliate

product:	key ingredients:	benefits:	results:

to protect your skin – a day cream

product:	key ingredients:	benefits:	results:

to repair and rebalance your skin – a night cream

product:	key ingredients:	benefits:	results:

specialized product recommendations

product:	key ingredients:	benefits:	results:

How to use your products

How to cleanse and tone

Cleanse

Apply to cupped hands, break down and smooth into face and neck with circular movements.

Remove with damp pads.

Tone

Apply toner to damp pads and smooth over entire area.

Always dry your skin after toning with a tissue.

How to exfoliate

Customize this wording to the products you sell.

Applying your day cream

Apply every morning after cleansing and toning.

Place a small amount of cream into hands, breakdown, then with gentle smoothing motions apply all over the face and neck.

Applying your night cream

Use night creams after cleansing and toning in the evening.

Warm up the balm/cream in the palm of the hands and apply using effleurage strokes to face and neck.

The smooth texture of the balm make it ideal for a mini massage to boost your skin.

Applying your specialized products

Customize this wording to the products you sell.

Your personal guide to building your range of …
(name of skin-care range)

_____

_____

_____

_____

_____

_____

_____

Recommended salon treatments

_____

_____

_____

_____

Next skin analysis

_____

_____

_____

_____

Please contact me personally if you
require further help and advice
on the ……………… product range.

Enjoy your products.

Selling is such an integral part of any salon

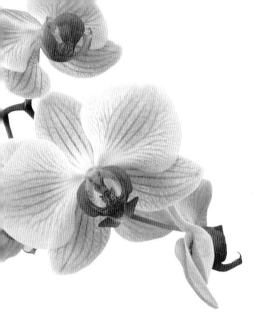

chapter seven
product knowledge

Introduction

Product knowledge still remains one of the corner-stones to professional selling. As the skin-care industry grows, the volume of products we offer to our clients is expanding at a rapid rate. As professional salespeople we must keep up to date regarding all existing products and new developments within the industry.

you will learn

Within this chapter we will review:

- How to identify products available for sale

- About the salon and legal requirements when selling

- About the importance of product knowledge to the sale

- How to remember essential product knowledge

Relevant Habia modules for NVQ Students: G4 and G11

 tip

Although effective and successful selling requires many more skills than product knowledge alone, it still remains one of the keys to achieving high level sales.

Using product knowledge to build trust with your clients

I am a passionate believer in product knowledge, it gives you, the salesperson, enormous self-confidence and you really feel professional when you know what you are talking about as opposed to waffling or bluffing. Excellent product knowledge gives you instant credibility and today's buyer will respect you if you have knowledge about what you are selling. It will also help build trust into the sales relationship.

Try selling something you know absolutely nothing about, not only is it very difficult and frustrating but your verbal communication will be broken, unrealistic and shoddy.

Today's buyers have a better understanding about what they are purchasing, they also have a greater power of choice than ever before. Excellent product knowledge can be the swing factor when clients have choice. The more your clients know about your products, the more they will think about them and focus on the benefits.

 tip

so what?

- Whenever you mention an ingredient or feature of a product always think to yourself, so what? because that is what your clients will be thinking.
- It is essential you add on the benefits to that feature and link the results to your clients' needs.

Product knowledge is not power, it is only potential power, it has to be applied correctly. For instance, if you say, 'This eye product contains hyaluronic acid' it will mean nothing to your clients until you add on that, 'this ingredient boosts hydration and plumps out the fine lines around eyes leaving the area moisturized and giving it a much more youthful appearance'.

Whilst most companies mistake product knowledge for sales training (the two are very different) most company trainers are like encyclopaedias for product information. Over the years I have experienced many trainers who have an excellent and thorough product knowledge. These people are great not only for initially teaching you about the products but also to engage in refresher training.

 tip

At least once a year have a product training day with the company's best trainer, absorb all the latest information and ask as many questions as possible.

The degree of product knowledge clients require varies immensely and at some point we have all been asked a question we simply could not answer. In this situation apologize and explain you will find the information as soon as possible. Never make up your answer: your clients will see through this and the trust bond will weaken and a sale could be lost.

> excellent product knowledge enhances your persuasive skills, builds trust and is a key part of successful selling

Professional knowledge

Professional knowledge is all the facts you know about the skin, body, nails, etc. We will have learnt all this information during our initial training, through continual education, from attending courses and reading trade journals.

We tend to take our professional knowledge for granted and yet it is an extremely powerful sales tool.

For example:

Professional knowledge point: the skin around the eyes is only one cell thick and due to this structure it is unable to absorb regular face creams.

Sales tool: Specially formulated eye creams can treat the area effectively. Their unique formulation allows the product to effectively penetrate this delicate area.

OR:

Professional knowledge point: The skin is continually shedding dead skin cells which can build up on the surface of the skin.

Sales tool: By using a skin exfoliator regularly you can remove this build-up and leave your skin looking radiant.

> Always keep the points simple and easy to understand or they will lose their impact.

Features and benefits

As I have already discussed people buy results, they buy what they think and feel the product will do for them. In order for clients to understand this, the therapist has to provide clear information about their products.

When prescribing products you need to discuss the features, benefits and results of the product. Always focus more on the benefits and the product results as this is what will influence the buying decision. More importantly, always link product benefits and results to clients' needs.

For example, during the consultation your clients may tell you they always apply a cream in the morning but by lunch time their skin feels dry again. This is obviously a concern for your clients so firstly select the correct product to treat it. Then during the presentation focus on the unique formulation of this product that allows moisture to be maintained in the skin, almost like a moisture reservoir. Mention this benefit first and then continue to discuss other relevant benefits.

> Clients tend to remember the first product benefit you mention so ensure it is a powerful one and one they personally need.

FAB

A lot of sales training uses the word FAB when teaching the relevance of features and benefits.

F = Features – the product ingredients
A = Attributes – what the features are doing
B = Benefits – what the features and attributes will do

This training technique is excellent, the word FAB is easy to remember. Over the years I have slightly tweaked this concept. People buy results and sometimes you can focus on the individual benefits at the cost of the overall result that clients will receive. This new development ensures you focus not only on the benefits, but more importantly, on the results.

F = Features – the product ingredients
A = Attributes – the exact action of the feature
B = Benefits – what the feature will do
R = Results – the overall results that benefit will give

Now the two concepts are very similar, almost identical, yet the difference in their outcome is powerful. Let's look at the application of each concept. The product I shall use for the example is an exfoliator which contains micro beads of brown sea algae.

FAB

Feature = brown sea algae
Attribute = gently removes dead skin cells
Benefits = the skin is left clearer and smoother

FAB+ R

Feature = brown sea algae
Attributes = gently removes dead skin cells
Benefits = the skin is left clearer and smoother
Results = the skin's texture is revived and regains its natural radiance. The effectiveness of your other skin-care products will be enhanced as they will penetrate deeper in to the skin.

By adding the 'R' you have to think a little more. You are simply explaining more benefits and in more detail to your clients. You almost have to expand the explanation and by doing so are more likely to encourage your clients to buy.

Remembering product knowledge

As the skin-care industry grows the volume of products in each range keeps increasing consequently we can be faced with at least 50 different products to remember and at most over 300. Trying to remember all the ingredients and actions for each product seems so daunting that it is enough to ensure many therapists never open their product training file again. However, by using a simple yet effective technique enough information about each product can be instantly accessed and eventually remembered to rapidly increase your sales. Initially this technique may take a little time, but it is a time investment well spent.

Creating a product information chart

A product information chart is an excellent way to ensure that all the key points about each and every product are recorded and easily accessed. This chart will prove indispensable when completing your clients' prescription guide. The chart is an excellent revision tool and is great to use for sales training. Once completed it is best presented on A4 laminated sheets. Initially time consuming, but once completed only new products or small amendments need ever be added.

Action – 15 minutes to excellent product knowledge

To create this chart you will need to spend 15 minutes per day collecting and adding all the relevant information. We can all find 15 minutes, just cut down on the amount of television you watch, get up a little earlier or utilize those spaces in your appointment book. To accelerate the production of your chart focus on three to five products each day. The quicker you complete this chart the faster your sales levels will increase.

1 Choose a retail product, always start with the most popular products your sell, e.g. cleansers, toners, moisturizers.

my biggest ever sale!

Selling the benefits is so powerful that if you really and passionately believe in something you can sell it (as long as your clients need or desire it).

Sixteen years ago I fulfilled a life-long goal to go on a cruise holiday. Ever since I can remember it was always my dream holiday. I went on a luxury cruise liner to the Caribbean with my parents and my sister and it truly was the holiday of a lifetime.

When I returned to work many of my clients asked all about my holiday, but one client in particular took a keen interest. She revealed that she too had always liked the idea of going on a cruise. So I began to tell her more about it, in other words I was selling the benefits. I passionately recalled the entire experience from departure to return.

Four weeks later the same client returned to the salon and during her treatment she excitedly explained that her husband and she had booked to go on the exact same cruise. They had, however, reserved a suite on board as they really were determined to enjoy their holiday of a lifetime. I can remember asking my client what made them book the holiday and to this day I can recall her response; 'After what you said about the cruise I went straight home to tell my husband all about it and there and then we telephoned the cruise agent and booked it!'

The cost of their holiday was £4,000, a lot of money today and definitely a lot of money then … and I had sold it to them.

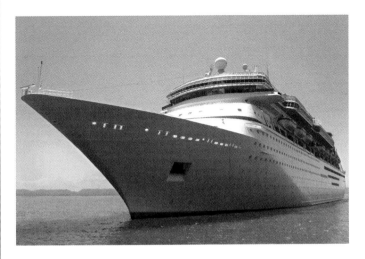

If you passionately believe in something you can sell it

2 By referring to your training file or the product packaging select two to three key ingredients (preferably ones you understand and can pronounce). These are features.

3 Select three key benefits of the product (Actions).

4 Choose the main result the product will give.

Then with this information fill in your chart.

Sample of chart

PRODUCT	INGREDIENTS	ACTIONS	RESULTS

For example:

PRODUCT	INGREDIENTS	ACTIONS	RESULTS
Moisturizing day cream	Hyaluronic acid sun filter SPF8	Drip feeds moisture into skin Plumps out fine lines Protects skin against sun damage	Skin feels continually hydrated and looks radiant Skin is protected from premature ageing by the sun

The key to this chart is to keep it simple and easy to follow. Because they are your words and you have created it you are more likely to utilize it and remember it. Only pick the recommended number of ingredients and actions to get to the essence of each product. This technique will not only ensure that your knowledge and passion will increase on a daily basis, but it will get you to focus on retail products.

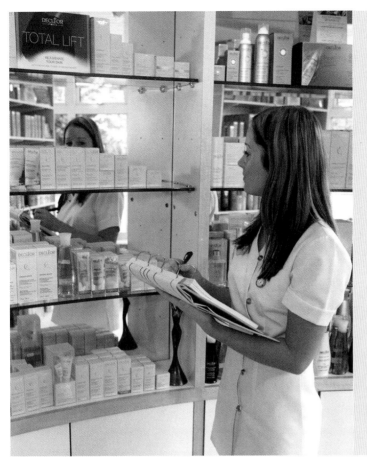

A product information chart is an excellent sales training and revision tool

After completion you now have an indispensable tool which you keep with you at all times at work and to use at home to revise. At a glance you can access information about each product, enough to use successfully in the sales process.

The product brochures that the skin-care houses produce for your clients are excellent revision tools. As a rule they have the key points regarding each product explained in a concise manner that will encourage clients to buy.

Extra techniques for remembering product knowledge

Visualization or using memory pegs

Within your salon you may have a selection of products which you sell regularly and therefore it is a great idea to be able to recall extra features and benefits of these products to increase the volume you sell, especially if their cost is high. Select between 5 and ten products which you sell on a consistent basis and with each one create a story or picture in your mind which will give a vivid description of your products' key ingredients, benefits and results. By using this visualization technique you will not only be able to remember an enormous amount of information about these popular products, but you will be able to access it rapidly for years to come. It is amazing how your mind remembers pictures and stories. The stranger the story or the image the more likely you are to remember it. Let me give you an example of this technique. I know this sounds a little strange, but I promise you it works. At the salon we sell a moisturizing cream – below I have listed the features and benefits as found in the product literature.

Ingredients	Benefits/results
Codium – a sea algae	Drip feeds the skin continuously, like a tap hydrating all the time
Papaya – melon	Removes dead skin cells by gently exfoliating – leaves skin radiant
Lavender	Calms and soothes the skin
Alginates – an amino acid	Traps water in cells
Extract of mushroom	Prevents water loss from the skin
Cassia – an exotic flower	Softens the appearance of fine lines

The picture I immediately visualize when I think of this product is (now wait for it, I said it will be strange!):

A person is walking on a beach and the sea is being filled by a dripping tap. This person walks into a hole in the sand which is filled with water and they get trapped. They are eating a melon and are holding a really big mushroom. They notice some lavender on the beach and next to it is a beautiful soft flower.

Now this story would mean nothing to anyone else but myself, but this is key for this technique to work. It has to be personal, you have to create it or you will forget it. Each part of the story automatically triggers my memory and I can recall what each part means, for instance *a hole in the sand* I remember is the ingredient alginate which traps water into the skin. Initially you have to have studied the product thoroughly in order for each picture to trigger your memory, for example, I know the action of lavender on the skin. Strange but true and effective is the best way to describe this visualization technique and once you have mastered this process it becomes effective and really good fun. It is also an excellent way to remember information about a new product or a product that is quite technical. Just give this technique a go, I will guarantee you will be amazed how effective it is.

Concept selling points

Concept selling points help you develop a clear concept about the products you retail and can be used to introduce the range generally, or they can be applied during the sales process. For each range of products you retail in your salon (for example skin-care, nail-care, make-up etc.) develop three overall concept selling points which encapsulate the benefits and facts about the range. For your skin-care range three concept selling points could be:

1 This unique range was developed 30 years ago and has attracted an unrivalled following of devoted clients.

2 It offers exceptional skin-care products which are designed to meet individual needs and deliver outstanding results.

3 The success of the range lies in the combination of technology and nature and the company's commitment to continually research and develop the most result-orientated products on the market today.

tip

> A great idea is to have your concept sale points printed on eye catching signs and placed in the staff room to act as a constant reminder to yourself and your team.

Group products together

Within most ranges you will notice similarities between product ingredients and therefore benefits. When this occurs you can group these products together and learn the key points that will enable you to rapidly increase your knowledge. Most ranges are divided into skin types or body concerns and by understanding the key points for each part of the range as a whole you will then be able to apply your knowledge to each different product when required. For example, the products designed for oily or combination skin could be a cleanser, toner, mask, treatment day cream and night cream. The key ingredients of all products could be tea tree, camphor and lavender. Learn the basic ingredients and their actions then adapt this knowledge according to the product function.

Mind maps

A great technique for training is to develop a mind map for product knowledge. This is a very simple technique but one that will give quick and outstanding results. The concept is to develop a chart or diagram of the product information as opposed to writing a list. The mind is more receptive to a picture and you are more likely to remember the key product benefits and features by using this technique. An example is shown below.

Mind maps are excellent tools for training and are indispensable for revision of existing products or initial training of new products. If possible use coloured pens when drawing them and by adding pictures their power will be amazing. Always display the mind maps in the team room and encourage each therapist to create their own.

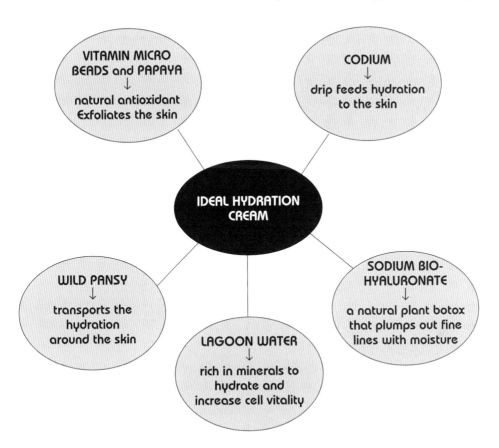

Labelled knowledge

Perhaps one of the oldest techniques we use is to label all our salon products that we use during treatments. Whilst they have their ingredients already printed on them, they can sometimes appear too detailed so we prefer to create our own bullet points by writing them on a white self adhesive sticker and placing them on the back of the product. It is also useful to write two or three benefits of the product on the label as well. Next time your clients comments on the aroma or ask what is in the product you are applying all the answers are there right in front of you.

This technique also enables you to read the key ingredients and benefits as you are performing a facial. Great revision!

Legal requirements

As professional salespeople it is essential that we provide our customers with accurate product information. Not only does this make commercial sense but it is also a legal requirement. There are two Acts of Parliament it is essential you are aware of.

Sale of goods act 1979

Essentially, this Act states that what you sell must fit its description, be fit for its purpose and be of satisfactory quality. If not, you – as the supplier – are obliged to sort out the problem.

Trades description act 1968

This Act makes it an offence if a trader:

a applies a false trade description to any goods; or

b supplies or offers to supply any goods to which a false trades description is applied; or

c makes certain kinds of false statement about the provision of any service.

✔ **key** reminders

- Knowing all about your products will increase the number of sales you close.

- By creating a product information chart you will rapidly increase your product knowledge.

- Create stories using visualization to remember product knowledge.

- Concept selling points are very effective and persuasive when used during the selling process.

Exercises

1 a Make a copy of the product information chart.
  b Select five retail products.
  c Taking one product at a time, fill in the chart. DO IT NOW!

Build your product chart daily – once completed your sales will grow.

2 Select a retail product.

- List all the features and benefits.

- Now, in your mind, create or visualize a story that encapsulates all the benefits of the product. Remember, the stranger the better.

- Repeat this visualization in your mind at least five times.

This system is fun and really works!

3 Create a 'mind map' for one retail product.

Create time to sell

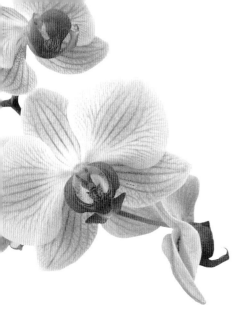

chapter eight

overcoming
objections

Introduction

Beauty therapy is a customer-focused business. We devote much time to customer care and rightly so, even to the extent that we welcome customer complaints. We not only learn from our mistakes but see them as an opportunity to improve our customer care policy, as clients are giving us information to help improve our service. Now take these points and relate them to selling. Think of objections as clients requesting extra information or reassurance that their needs will be met. Handling objections well is part of giving excellent customer care. When you take this approach you will welcome objections just as much as you welcome client comments.

you will learn

Within this chapter we will review:

- What an objection actually is
- Types of objections
- How to effectively handle price objections
- Why people don't buy
- Lost sales analysis – why you may not be achieving your sales

Relevant Habia modules for NVQ students: Unit G6

 tip

In selling if your clients say nothing it is pretty difficult to keep the conversation and sales process going. An objection is a great focal point to lead to a sale and handling objections professionally and efficiently will help you close the sale.

Two major types of objections

Genuine objections

The genuine objection is where clients are asking a sincere question about your product. You may not have clarified all the benefits or your clients may not have understood some of the information, either way you must take responsibility and recap the benefits, product application or results. It is vital to give all the relevant information to make your clients' buying decision easier. A genuine objection is logical: your clients' objections are real.

False objections

False objections do happen. Clients will raise a point which clearly shows they do not wish to purchase your products. If this situation occurs regularly you need to ask yourself a series of questions:

1 Are you qualifying your clients correctly?

2 Have you created desire to purchase your products?

3 Are you linking your product benefits to your clients' concerns?

4 Are you selling the results?

In reality we will all face false objections even when we answer yes to all the above questions. Sometimes the sale is just not going to happen; refrain from being pushy or appear desperate. You want your clients to return to your salon, leave the door open.

> Objections could simply be the way your clients slow down the sales process. They may need time to think before they buy.

✔ **tip**

- When I recognize a client is not going to buy, I say how much I have enjoyed helping them with their skin-care.

- I then proceed to give them a couple of samples but then (and this is very important), I spend some time showing the client how to use them.

- I am still focusing on relationship selling. The result is the client leaves feeling valued and will return.

- The client feels happy with the service and I learn from that sales experience because …

- When they return to the salon I can begin the sales process again.

Some other types of objections

There are many objections your clients could raise during the sales process:

- size of the product

- product texture

- product packaging (glass as opposed to plastic)

- price

- product aroma

- the home-care recommendations seem too complicated.

When your clients raise objections to the sale, ensure you completely understand it, if necessary ask more questions to find out exactly what they mean. Always respect your clients' objections, never dismiss them. If your clients have a genuine objection it must be important to them.

In order for the sale to proceed clients must feel you answered their objection.

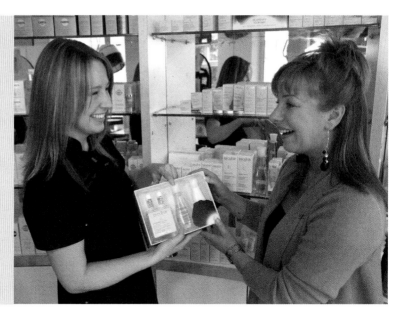

Handling objections well is part of giving excellent customer care

Let's talk price

I feel the need to mention the subject of price in greater detail as it is the one objection many therapists say is the reason they do not achieve their sales potential. I think subconsciously therapists view price as something out of their control so it can never be overcome. Let's examine this issue of price.

You will always have clients who desire to pay a lot for skin-care, whilst other clients aim to pay as little as possible. During the consultation you must ascertain which products your clients have previously purchased. This will act as a guide as to how much they are used to spending on skin-care. If you are selling professional salon products to your clients but they are not used to spending on a good skin-care range, then price could be an issue. Always be prepared for price objections as they will occur. Below are a few tips to help overcome them.

- If your clients say, 'This product sounds really good but it is too expensive'. Your response could be, 'I can understand your concern about the price. Many clients indeed felt the same way, yet after using the product for a few days they were so pleased at the results they say it was worth the investment.' In this example you are showing empathy towards your clients' price objections. Your response explains that your clients are not alone in initially thinking the price is too high. Yet the benefits outweigh the price of the product and the results justify it.

- The words you speak are vital; instead of 'buying' choose 'investment'. For example, 'this product is a great investment for your skin'. With an investment you get something back; it provokes a better way of thinking.

- Sell the difference. This is one of my favourites. If your clients usually spend £20 on a day cream and the one you are recommending is £35 then simply sell the difference. An example would be, 'For just £15 the added benefits are an SPF15 to protect your skin from the sun's harmful rays, an amazing texture that melts into your skin', and so on.

- Break the price down in to small units. If a product is priced as £50 and lasts 12 weeks, the cost per week is £4.16, the daily cost only 60 pence – now that sounds affordable.

- Say its value. If asked the price, instead of saying 'it costs £50' say 'its value is £50'.

a dictionary definition of cost is:

'have as its price; involve the sacrifice or loss of'

a dictionary definition of value is:

'the amount of money something is worth, the importance or usefulness of something'

It may "cost" you not to remember the "value" of these two definitions. Having kept this in mind, then present the client with more information.

for example:

'Its value is £50 for a 50ml jar which can be used every day and will last three months.'

The client will not only hear the price but the benefits and facts about her purchase.

- How you view the price will have an impact on how your clients see and feel about it. Believe it or not many products we sell are reasonably priced. Take a walk around that department store again: you may be surprised at the amount of money people are willing to spend on beauty products. If price is an issue to you then this will be passed on to your clients. When selling, I always mention that our products are a premium skin-care range.

> As beauty therapists we are offering a professional service, backed with extensive training, national qualifications, years of experience all wrapped up with great customer care – we are offering a good deal. Be proud of the price and this positivity will pass to your clients.

- If you really want something, price is rarely an issue. Be sure to focus on the benefits and results your product will deliver, sell the dream and add the passion and conviction that your products are perfect for your clients.

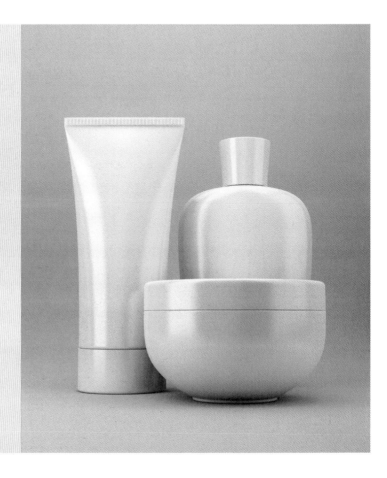

Clients will pay more for products if you convince them they're good value

Is price really the issue?

People do not necessarily want the cheapest or the most expensive product, what they require is value for money. Realistically clients want the best products with the lowest amount of risk. Try this experiment:

Present three suitable products to your clients, they must perform the same function (for example, they should all be cleansers), the only difference between the three must be the price. So you may have:

Cleanser A	£ 8.00
Cleanser B	£17.00
Cleanser C	£28.00

A few clients may choose cleanser A and a few cleanser C but the majority will purchase cleanser B, why? Because it presents the best value for money with a low risk.

When recommending products, always try to give your clients a choice, people enjoy being given options it helps them feel in control of their purchasing decision.

 tip

Always give clients a choice of products that they could purchase.

When I introduced a new expensive skin-care range in to the salon, it was amazing how the sales of our existing less expensive range increased. The reasons for this were two-fold. Firstly, when the client was recommended products from our existing range and then the new range, they perceived the former as affordable with less risk. Secondly, the therapists' approach changed as they too viewed a product priced at £56 good value compared to its compatible product from our new range priced at £110. In reality all that had changed was the clients' and therapists' perception of the product prices.

If you lower your clients' perception of risk you will close more sales.

 tip

Never use the word 'cheap' when referring to the price, instead use the word 'inexpensive'.

 real life example

my worst ever sale!

Recently a client visited the salon for a facial treatment. The main reason for her visit was to combat the exceptionally dry and rough skin on her face. As I began the consultation she informed me she was getting married in seven days! To add to this dilemma I was doing her wedding make-up! The client lived abroad and her mother, who was a regular client of the salon, had simply booked all her appointments for the week before the wedding so we had not been given the opportunity to perform a wedding consultation any earlier. My client informed me that she worked outdoors and never used any skin-care products; this was reflected in the skin condition I was now faced with. There was absolutely no way her wedding make-up would be successfully applied to her skin as it was at present.

In my opinion I had no choice but to recommend a selection of products that she would have to use intensely at home for the next seven days. My client agreed to follow a routine, so after her treatment, I began the product advice and she agreed

to take them all: we both felt there was no option.

My aim was to get the best improvement with her skin in the shortest possible time; her skin requirements were at the heart of my recommendations. However, in my speed to deal with this dilemma, I had at no point mentioned the price of the products. Imagine my client's reaction; remember she never purchases skin care products, when her bill came to £152. Talk about client objections!

My mistake was I had not price conditioned my client. She had no idea the cost of premium skin-care products; I should have introduced their cost at a much earlier stage and handled her objections then. As it happened she was now stood at the reception desk holding a carrier bag with the products already inside! I have never forgotten this experience as it taught me a very valuable lesson which I call price conditioning.

Back to my client, £152 worth of products and one very embarrassed therapist. The client's response was not 'I cannot afford them', her actual words were 'How much? £152 for skin creams!' Luckily (for me anyway) the client's mother was sitting

real life example continued

in the reception area and immediately said to her daughter that she would pay the bill.

I wrote this case study reluctantly and with reservations, but it shows that we all make mistakes, regardless of experience. The key is always to learn from our errors and never knowingly repeat them again.

Always 'price condition' your clients to avoid nasty surprises

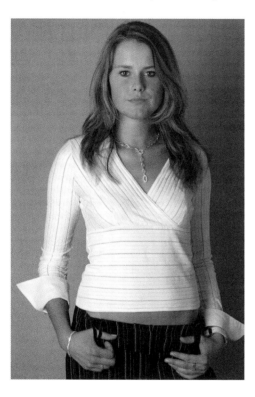

Why people don't buy

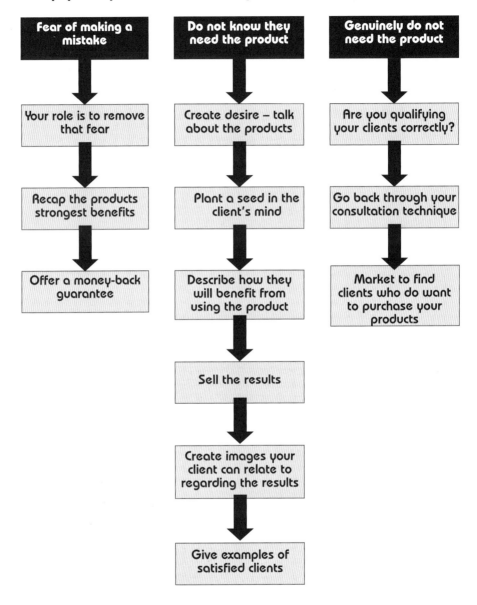

The above charts shows the three main reasons a client will not buy.

The first reason

Fear of making a mistake. Your clients may have made many purchases in the past that they may later have regretted. They probably want the product but are afraid of making that final decision. Ensure you recap the benefits and focus on the results they will receive from using the product. I have personally found the best way to sell to clients who have a real fear of making a mistake is to offer a money-back guarantee, or the choice of swapping the product if they are not satisfied. Naturally you must check whether this is adhering to salon policy before you offer clients this guarantee.

I have been offering this money-back guarantee for many years now and usually only have a few products a year returned.

The second reason

Clients do not know they need the product. This reason can take a little longer to overcome. Through educating your clients on the importance and benefits of using a professional salon range, you will begin to plant a seed in their mind about using the products. Again focus on the benefits and give testimonials of satisfied clients who have used the product.

The third reason

They genuinely do not need the product. Never try to sell a product to a client if they do not need it.

Lost sales analysis

If you are losing more sales than you are achieving, look through the checklist below. It highlights the main reasons sales are lost. The list will help you pinpoint the areas you will need to focus on to put your sales back on track.

1 Failure to establish rapport with your clients.

2 Not transferring enough passion and enthusiasm.

3 Poor product demonstration.

4 Not focusing on product results.

5 Failure to link product benefits to your client's exact needs.

6 Being too pushy.

7 Poor product knowledge.

8 Not asking the right questions.

9 Not actively listening to your clients.

10 Not offering clients a choice of retail products.

11 Failure to handle your clients' objections.

12 Failure to qualify clients correctly.

13 Not creating desire for your products.

14 Failure to ask for the sale.

15 Making wild claims about your products.

✔ **key** reminders

- Learn to welcome objections.
- Objections are usually the means clients will use to gain more information or clarification.
- Choose your words carefully.
- Always, always, give clients a choice of products.

Exercises

A client, with a skin concern, visits your salon for a consultation. After your recommendations they raise the following objections:

1 The products cost more than I am used to paying.

2 I will buy them another time.

3 I am already using similar products.

4 I think I will use up my existing products first.

Prepare an answer to overcome each objection (remember the client has a skin concern and her existing products are obviously not giving her results).

There is no failure in selling, just feedback

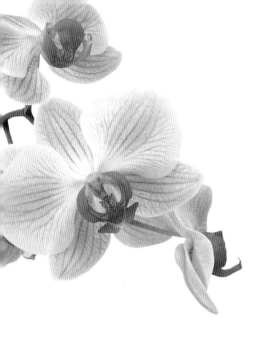

chapter nine
closing the sale

Introduction

Closing the sale is simply asking for the order. Many sales have been lost purely because they were not asked for. If you have followed a good sales procedure you will have established a rapport, asked questions and listened to understand your clients' needs. You will also have performed an excellent presentation, sold the benefits and results of the products and answered any questions to overcome their objections. The final stage is to ask for the sale. Easily done, closing the sale would be 'Which products would you like to take today?'

The reason most salespeople avoid this last stage is a fear of rejection; fear that clients might say 'no thank you'. This, however, is the worst outcome, three little words: 'no thank you'. Accept some sales will inevitably end in a 'no' – it is par for the course, move on and keep selling and closing.

you will learn

Within this chapter we will review:

- The importance of closing the sale
- How to close the sale
- When to close
- Why it is important to be confident during closing

Relevant HABIA modules for NVQ students: Unit G6

tip

By not asking for the sale you are not giving your clients the opportunity to buy and that is not fair.

The importance of closing a sale

You will lose 100 per cent of the sales you don't ask for. In my experience many sales are lost for four reasons:

1 Failure to qualify your clients and create a desire for your products: the clients were not ready to buy.

2 Clients may not realize their concerns. They may have been given a gift voucher and therefore their perception of the visit was as a treat. The chances are they have not even thought of home-care products.

3 Not having time to sell is probably the biggest reason many of us have not yet reached our sales potential. We are almost too busy to be successful salespeople. If you have not allowed yourself enough time to follow the steps that lead to a sale it is advisable to wait and avoid rushing a sale. Instead create the desire for your retail products and then either add on extra time during your clients' next treatments, or invite them back for a complementary mini treatment and consultation during which you can focus purely on their home-care routine.

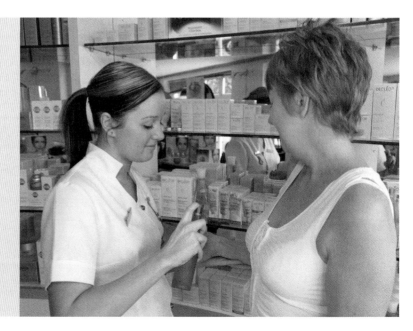

Always close the sale – you will lose 100 per cent of the sales you never asked for

4 The sale was not asked for. By not closing your sales or not asking for the sales you may subconsciously send the wrong messages to your clients. It may appear you are not 100 per cent convinced that they should purchase the products. Failure to close can show a lack of conviction on your part. Face your fear, closing is not that bad. Remember be positive about your recommendations, passionate about your products, focus on their benefits and wrap it all up in total belief that you have performed to a professional standard. Then ask for the sale.

How to close a sale

Closing questions

The best way to close a sale is to use a closing question or statement that is relevant and will be effective in the sales situation you are in. Below is a selection of closing questions you will find helpful. Choose the ones you feel comfortable and confident using.

'Which products would you like to take today?'

'Of your five key products which will you be purchasing today?'

'I want you to really notice a difference, by using this product, you will see a real improvement.'

'Will you be taking the 200ml cleanser or the 400ml?'

'Would you prefer the cream or the emulsion in this product?'

'This exfoliator is one of our top selling products, in fact we are down to our last one.'

'It is amazing how quickly these products are bought, as quick as we restock we sell out again.'

Shut up!

When you have asked your closing question wait for a reply. Your clients need time to think. Silence is golden; let your clients answer the question; a pause is a good buying signal. If you interrupt or answer the question yourself not only will you appear pushy but it may be interpreted as desperation for the sale, neither are ideals in selling.

Body language

When closing sales your body language is exceptionally important. The two most important actions are:

1 Smile

2 Maintain eye contact with your clients.

Both of these actions are very positive and will make your clients feel comfortable and encourage them to buy.

Buying signals

During the sales process, especially when closing, you should be constantly looking for buying signals from your clients. The three signals that I find the most encouraging are:

1 If clients ask a lot of questions regarding the products and your home-care advice.

2 When clients agree positively with the advice you are giving.

3 When clients are using positive body language, for example, smiling, maintaining eye contact, a relaxed posture, etc.

When to close

As a basic rule you always close towards the end of the sales process. However, in reality you can start to close very early in the sales process. For instance, during a consultation you could use an encouraging closing statement 'I know my products will help you tremendously, but first I need to ask you a few more questions'.

The key is to watch for buying signals which are your cue to start closing. The client may ask 'How often would I use the mask?' or 'When would I apply the eye cream? Clients may even ask for more details about the products.

Be confident during closing

All of these are showing an interest so start closing. Suggest they begin using a certain product immediately to help solve their concern, or show your clients the various retail sizes of the product. Use positive phrases and words to encourage your clients.

If you have given good service and excellent customer care closing will not only be easy, but natural and comfortable.

> ## if you don't close you don't sell

The golden minute

After each sale whether successful or not spend 60 seconds recording all the relevant information:

- the products you sold

- all the recommendations you gave

- any samples given

- general information which you need to remember for your client's next visit.

At your clients' next treatment you can ask how well the products are performing or if they enjoyed using the samples. Again, you are focusing on relationship selling, even a few weeks after the sale demonstrating you still care.

✔ key reminders

- Closing the sale is simply asking for the order.

- You will lose 100 per cent of the sales you do not ask for.

- Have to hand a selection of closing questions that you can use naturally and effectively.

- When you have asked for the sale – SHUT UP – let your client think and respond.

real life example

the client who will never buy

It is inevitable that some people will never buy from you. In our industry people tend to initially come to the salon for treatments and retailing is a service we introduce to them once they have arrived. As I mentioned previously, many therapists have this as their reason for low retail sales, they too see themselves only as treatment providers. After applying both your new psychology of selling and your new sales techniques, you would think that all clients would follow your recommendations and purchase products, but this is not always the case.

A client of mine has a severely sensitive and reactive skin which causes her great discomfort. I have tried every approach to encourage her to purchase the products that I confidently know will help her skin, but to no avail.

During one visit I decided to conduct a sales experiment. After her treatment I prescribed the products and received the usual reaction which was that she was happy with her existing range (which obviously was not working). My experiment was to try a new kind of closing technique. I suggested she took all the products home to try and return them at her next appointment in four weeks and, wait for this, she did not have to pay for them. Simply take them, try them and then return them, no charge. Warning – do not try this at home, sorry salon! This was a deliberate exercise which I carried out purely for my sales research, and I knew the client and her family very well. The response from my client was astounding, she declined my offer, she did not want to take the products.

In the future she may well follow my recommendations, I do hope so. If your closing techniques do not work do not get pushy, sometimes your clients are just not going to buy no matter what you are offering.

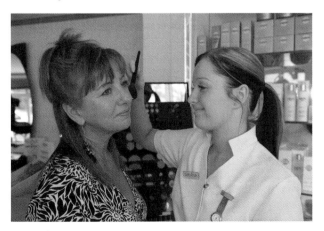

Never get pushy, even if you are having trouble closing a sale

Exercises

Select three closing questions that you feel comfortable asking. Write them on a separate card and keep them with you to act as a constant reminder of how easy it is to ask for the sale.

Thinking about selling is not enough, you must take ACTION

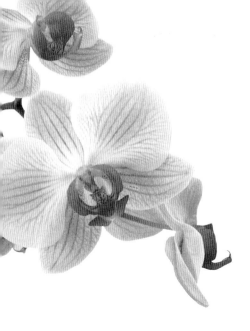

techniques and aids to help you sell

Introduction

People believe what they see. Of all the senses vision is the most powerful so take this fact on board when selling. By using visual aids during the sales process you will greatly enhance your sales figures.

Below are three tools that may seem very simple in concept yet will provide remarkable results. As with all my suggestions, all I ask is that you give them a try.

you will learn

Within this chapter we will review:

- How the use of practical tools will increase your sales figures
- How by adopting professional and caring techniques you will close more sales

The 'beautiful selling' prescription guide

This is a powerful tool that when used correctly and effectively will dramatically increase your sales. The procedure is discussed in detail in Chapter 6 on product presentation and demonstration; to recap on the benefits:

- it is personalized to each client
- it demonstrates you have devoted time to your clients' concerns
- it names the products, their key ingredients and benefits and the results they will give
- it shows how to use each product correctly – client education
- it advises which products to purchase first
- it recommends suitable treatments – link selling.

All wrapped up with your personal and caring touch.

Skin chart

Skin charts are a coloured picture showing the cross-section of the skin and are available from most beauty product wholesalers. This effective diagram shows the three layers of skin and the benefits of using it during the sales presentation are truly amazing. This tool enables you to take an expert and professional approach to skin-care and allows you to use your knowledge and training. As you explain the product benefits to your clients you can use the diagram to show how and where the products work, almost like action points on the chart. The diagram will clearly show and explain the advice you are giving. For example you can clearly explain where the products work in reference to the skin layers. Through visual interaction your clients' understanding will be increased. As you present each product you refer to your chart and explain which layer of skin it is treating, why it is important to treat that layer and the results your product will give.

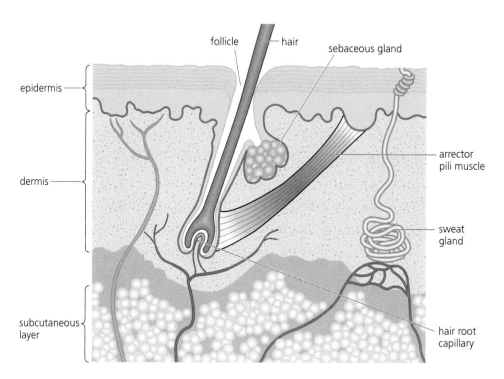

using the skin chart when selling

The first time I used a skin chart during the sales process was quite by accident. My previous client was a new client for electrolysis and I had used the chart to explain the hair growth cycle. During the product recommendations with my next client, I was explaining the cause of her oily skin

and noticed I had left the chart on my trolley. I simply used it to demonstrate the role of the sebaceous glands, but found my client's interest in what I was saying increased. She was pointing to the chart and asking questions, good buying signals. Not all clients will be interested to that degree but you may be pleasantly surprised how many are.

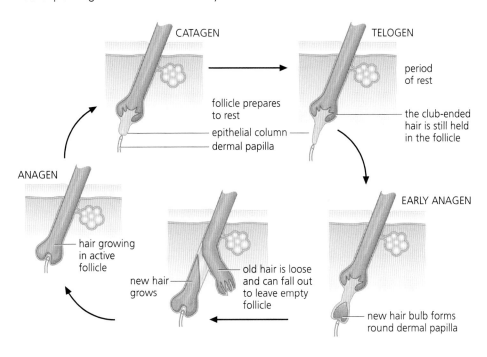

CATAGEN

TELOGEN

period of rest

follicle prepares to rest
epithelial column
dermal papilla

the club-ended hair is still held in the follicle

ANAGEN

EARLY ANAGEN

hair growing in active follicle

new hair grows

old hair is loose and can fall out to leave empty follicle

new hair bulb forms round dermal papilla

Compliment slips

A bookshop I frequent started putting a small compliment slip in their books to thank you for shopping at their book store; as I open the book even though I know they always put a slip in, it is so nice when I find it. By placing a similar compliment slip in with your clients' purchases the same effect will be achieved when they arrive home and open their bags. A simple pre-printed message on a card or paper slip has a great impact, for example:

> Thankyou for your custom
>
>   Ruth.x.

Or

> It has been my pleasure to serve you
>
>   Ruth.x.

It is always the little things you do that will have the greatest impact. I remember 16 years ago I took my first flight with Virgin Atlantic and during the in-flight movie we were served with an ice cream. I thought that was such a fantastic thing to do, at the time no other airline was focusing on the little service details. I cannot remember how smooth the flight was or whether it was on schedule, I just remember how good it felt to be offered the ice cream, it was different.

 tip

- To achieve success it is important to model success.
- Many of the world's most successful companies are client focused, they always have an attitude of gratitude and think service, service, service!

✔ **key** reminders

- The use of a bespoke prescription guide will immediately increase your retail sales whilst enhancing your customer service.

- The use of a skin-care chart will demonstrate your professional knowledge and reinforce your recommendations.

- The little touches, e.g. compliment slips, do make a difference, implement as many as you can.

Exercises

Two very simple tasks, but do them now.

1 Order a skin chart for yourself. Either place on the treatment room wall or keep on your trolley. If it has been a while since you were at college, study the chart, refer back to your training to refamiliarize yourself with it. Then use it during the next consultation and product presentation.

2 Design your own compliment slip and print a few to use immediately.

If you believe you are a poor salesperson, or a great salesperson, you are probably right. Develop a positive mental attitude

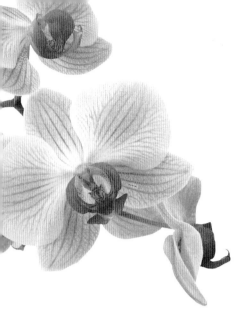

promotions to increase retail sales

Introduction

From time to time we all need a little boost to help increase our level of sales and reach or indeed exceed our target. With so much competition out there from the stores, shopping channels and even other salons we have to be proactive and seek out new and exciting ways to achieve more sales. Below is a selection of ideas to increase your sales. The list is endless and the more you focus on finding new ways to promote your products, the more you will develop new and exciting ways to do so.

you will learn

Within this chapter we will review:

- The importance of planning and implementing various activities to increase sales levels
- How to inform clients about additional products and services that are available
- How selling will contribute to the financial effectiveness of the business

Relevant Habia modules for NVQ students: Unit G6, Unit BT10 and Unit G11

Planning a retail promotion

All retail promotions should focus on developing and growing your retail sales. Their aim should always be to help build a strong retail culture in the salon.

The retail promotion must benefit:

1 The salon – the promotion must be a good marketing idea to increase retail sales. Try to choose a popular retail product, one that is generic and that will benefit the majority of clients. The promotion should also benefit the salon financially even if a money-off promotion is in place.

2 The client – the promotion should appeal to clients and be tempting to try.

3 The therapist – will therapists enjoy promoting this product or service? A good idea is to ask and encourage the team to assist in the development of promotions.

Gift with purchase

Within department stores gift with purchase (GWP) is one of the best ways to attract and increase retail sales. The GWP promotion has always been a firm favourite of mine and prior to my suppliers offering this type of promotion I would create my own gifts. Clients love receiving a free gift and GWP will really increase your sales because:

- It is a great way to introduce retail to clients by showing the free gift currently available; therapists love to give their clients a free gift almost as much as the clients love receiving them.

- You feel confident and positive selling your products as you are working by the principle of always giving people more than they expect to get.

- It provides a great talking point to clients, a positive way to introduce retail.

- It encourages clients to buy your products.

- For the nervous or inexperienced sales person, GWP always seems to help them retail more.

Skin consultation days

Although most salons offer complimentary skin care consultations what we tend to find is that clients generally book in for treatments first. A good way to increase your level of skin consultations, which will directly lead to an increase in retail sales, is to hold special days where clients are invited to experience a mini treatment and a complete skin consultation with a home-care programme. Whether you charge for the treatment (usually a booking fee) or not is up to you. If you choose to, it may be a good idea to redeem the cost against any purchases. The focus of this promotion is not the treatment but your clients' skin-care and home-care requirements, therefore the treatment should only take about 30 minutes and aim to include a cleanse, exfoliation, mask application and moisturize. The aim of the treatment is to introduce products and techniques to your clients so think of it as almost a demonstration. Avoid a long facial massage as this can then become too similar to a treatment. Your clients will feel and see how amazing their skin is during and after. Talk through what you are doing, why and how great their skin is responding to the product applications. If clients usually purchase their products from shops or chemists then they will be totally impressed by your technique, knowledge and professionalism.

Skin consultation days can be held as often as required, but follow these few guidelines for maximum success:

- Hold them on normally quiet days of the week.

- Promote and hold them during quiet times of the year for instance January and November.

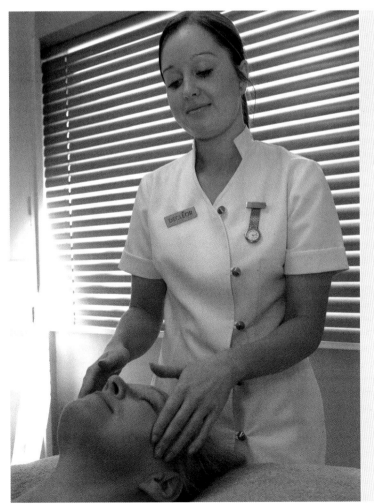

Offering complementary skin care consultations is a good way to increase sales

- Allow plenty of time for each client, this is an opportunity for you to have time to sell which may not be available during your usual busy day.

- Effective promotion prior to these days is essential. Market them in your salon by word of mouth, leaflets and posters, mail shot existing clients with a personal invitation or even simply telephone a selection of clients and invite them to enjoy a complimentary treatment with home-care advice. Alternatively, you can advertise on the ladies page of your local newspaper to attract new clients, consider inviting the editor to attend and experience the promotion.

Product focus promotions

This promotion is an amazing way to boost sales and best of all, once set up, requires little effort to run. The idea is to focus on one or two products for a period of time and promote them to as many clients as possible. Follow this easy technique and watch the sales follow:

- Select a product which can be used by most people, for example, hand cream, eye masks, body exfoliators, face exfoliators or body creams. If the product is too specific the promotion will not be as successful, it needs to appeal to the majority.

- Produce relevant literature in the form of a flyer to be able to hand out to your clients. Include the product benefits and results, client testimonials and any price promotion.

- Create an eye-catching display and ensure you have a good stock level of this promotional product. A word of caution regarding displays – never ever rely on them alone to communicate a message to your clients. The best example of this is when I gave birth to my son. My team created a blue display consisting of balloons, banners and a large congratulation sign in the reception. The amount of clients (especially regular ones) who once in the treatment room asked their therapist 'has Ruth had her baby yet?' taught me a valuable lesson. Displays play an important role but nothing replaces word of mouth. Good communication between two people will guarantee client awareness and is more likely to lead to a sale.

- You need to inform your team about the promotion and all the relevant information. Hold a product training session to cover the product's uses, ingredients, benefits, results, when and how to use the product and have testimonials about the product to motivate your team. Play some of my sales games to reinforce.

- The promotion can run for a minimum of one week to a maximum of four weeks or while stocks last' (a great quote to encourage your clients to buy now).

- Offer either a small amount of money off or buy one get one half price (great if you have over-purchased a particular product) or simply promote the product with no financial incentive.

Running product focus promotions encourages all the team to retail and gives them an easy opportunity to retail to many clients. You will find that by asking if they noticed the display in reception or by simply handing your clients the product information sheet you can comfortably initiate a conversation about home-care products and home-care advice.

Hold a 'beauty school' evening

This unique concept will not only increase your retail sales but also your client base. At least four times a year invite existing clients to an evening called 'beauty school'. Encourage your clients to bring a friend, preferably one that has never visited the salon before.

During the evening discuss the importance of home-care and demonstrate how to professionally and correctly:

- cleanse and tone

- exfoliate

- apply day cream, night cream and eye cream

- perform a home facial massage
- apply a face mask.

The entire evening should be devoted to how to look after your skin at home, how to use the products correctly and the benefits each stage will give your skin. Alternatively the focus of the evening could be body-care or nail-care.

You can either have one demonstration or several in a different treatment room each showing a different stage so that small groups of clients can flow from room to room to watch and learn each technique. What will surprise you is how many people have never been shown how to perform a professional skin-care routine.

your aim is to educate your clients

Help your clients achieve the best from their products, have extra therapists available to perform a personal skin consultation or book clients an appointment for one as soon as possible. During the beauty school evening you are not directly trying to sell but to educate clients. However, what will begin to happen is you create a desire and clients will begin to purchase products.

Don't forget customer care during the evening. Serve complimentary refreshments and nibbles to make the evening really enjoyable. A great touch is to give your clients a goodie bag containing a few product samples. Even add an individually boxed continental chocolate and by including a voucher for a percentage discount off a facial treatment you will increase your salon utilization levels.

The above examples are ways to help you personally improve your selling skills and sales. This book was never intended to cover all marketing ideas such as buy two products, get one free, or half price sale. These promotions have their place but as with any price reduction if you do it too often, clients will not only expect it, but also refrain from purchasing until your sale. Keep these price reductions to a minimum to avoid sending your clients the wrong message.

By implementing the product promotion ideas your focus will be kept on your retailing skills and can provide great motivation, keeping you on track to reach your target, especially during quiet times.

real life example

my most sucessful promotion

After 21 years in the beauty industry I have people who have been clients for many years. Consequently I feel the need to constantly create new treatments that will appeal to them without going to the expense of continually investing in new product ranges or expensive equipment.

I created a new facial treatment that involved the use of two key products. During the treatment these two products were promoted to my clients. The first was an exfoliator. As we applied the product all the benefits were explained to the clients and we even gave the clients a hand-held mirror so they could see the improvement after its application. The second product was a scrumptious creamy mask that was

used as the massage medium. Clients could feel their skin was amazingly soft and radiant after its application. During the treatment we focused heavily on these two products constantly selling the benefits.

After the treatment the clients were given special product literature about the two products. Their therapist advised on how to use the products at home and how they would easily slot in to their existing home-care routine.

To this day I am still amazed at the success of the promotion. It was a simple idea but it worked well. No financial incentive was offered, we sold at full retail price. Its success was due to the two products selected, the simplicity of the treatment and the passion, enthusiasm and product knowledge of the therapists.

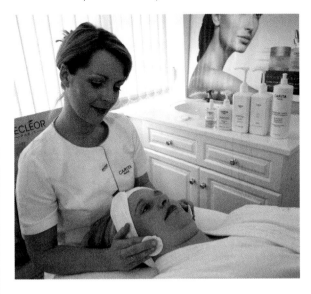

Educating your clients about the benefits of products will increase their desire to buy them

✔ **key** reminders

- By planning ahead your retail promotions can be evenly spaced throughout the calendar year.

- Offer various promotions but take care when reducing recommended retail prices.

- Become proactive with product promotions, do not just allow your products to just sit on the shelf.

Exercises

1 a Select one promotion, from the above examples, that you can begin within the next four weeks.

   b Develop an action plan, for example, dates for skin-care days, select products for a product focus promotion etc.

   c Implement your action plan immediately.

   d As always, monitor the results and success of the promotion.

2 In order to continually achieve good sales figures within the salon, it is essential you spend time planning a varied selection of promotions and activities to help you reach your targets. The most resourceful way to achieve this is to plan at least six months in advance. Take a yearly planner and for each month plan a retail promotion. Consider all the various activities you could offer to ensure a good variety will be offered in the salon or spa.

Thoughts control your actions... choose yours carefully

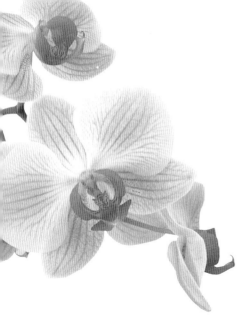

goal setting in selling

Introduction

Start dreaming

I believe in dreaming and having a vision. Many motivational speakers and coaches say that dreaming leads nowhere, instead have goals, goals, goals! Whilst I passionately believe in goal setting, I feel that it is the second stage. The first stage I have is a dream. I think about it and use visualization techniques to imagine how achieving my dream will make me feel. I spend quite a long time on stage one and if I develop such a passion towards it I develop it into a goal. I believe the dream gives the goal strength, as it gives it a burning desire to be achieved whilst giving you the determination for success that basic goal setting can sometimes omit.

> Those who dream by night, in the dusty recesses of their minds, wake to find it was all vanity. But the dreamers of the day are dangerous, for they may act their dreams with open eyes and make things happen.
>
> T. E. Lawrence

By purchasing this book you have a dream to fulfil your true sales potential. Now let's turn that dream into reality by using targets.

you will learn

Within this chapter we will review:

- How to reach your sales goals through the setting of targets: daily, weekly and monthly

- The power and importance of setting targets

- How your treatment mix can affect your level of sales

Relevant HABIA modules: Unit G8, Unit G11

Setting yourself targets

Success is achieved by taking small consistent steps towards your target or goal. This book will provide the steps, but it is up to you to take action to achieve success. By setting yourself targets you can assess your performance. Targets work best if they are achievable and with a little extra action on your part, they will then become motivational as you will see them as realistic. If your average weekly sales are £100 and you set yourself an immediate target of £500 this may be achievable in the long term, but initially it may well act as a demotivator. A new weekly target of £200 is more realistic in the near future and is therefore motivational. Your long-term target could be weekly sales of £1,000, but set yourself short-term targets and take small consistent steps to get you there. I agree anything is possible but time and experience are usually key factors in achieving high weekly sales on a consistent basis.

Treatment mix

I have a saying which is blunt but to the point, 'I know you can sell a skin care cream during a pedicure but it is a lot easier during a facial!' What I am saying is look at the treatment mix you are doing, then look at the volume of your sales. For example, if you spend most of your time doing treatments such as eyebrow trims, eyelash tints, underarm waxes, etc. your retail sales may be lower due to your treatment mix. Another reason is that many of these treatments involve less time being spent with your clients. When your clients book appointments for a facial treatment the chances are they are concerned with their skin. Creating the desire has almost taken care of itself, whilst your clients are having an under-

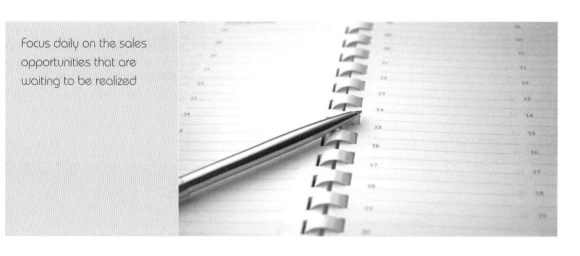

Focus daily on the sales opportunities that are waiting to be realized

arm wax they will be primarily concerned with hair removal and creating the desire for skin-care can take time. (I don't know about you but I find an under-arm wax can take as little as five minutes to perform.)

Whilst this book is not intended to be a guide on marketing, it may well be worth looking at the kind of treatments you are busiest with as a salon and con-sider attracting a higher percentage of face and body treatments. The teleshop-ping channels appeal to the right audience, as they market a one-hour beauty special and thousands of viewers tune in. What viewers is your salon attracting? What marketing could you do to get the right audience into your salon?

Setting daily targets

When you arrive at the salon tomorrow, instead of looking at your appointments to see how busy you are or if you have a lunch break (yes we all do it!), look instead for sales opportunities instead.

Ask yourself the following questions:

- What treatments have I got today?
- Which of these, if I applied a little effort, could lead to a sale?
- Are there any new clients in?
- Which existing clients have not purchased for a while?
- Which existing clients have never purchased? (Yes, we all have them.)

Begin to think Sales! Sales! Sales! Depending on your answers, set yourself a target. If you have many finishing touch treatments like waxing or lash tints you may set a target of £100. The next day your treatment mix may involve three facials, one body treatment and two new clients for skin-care advice, in this case your daily target may be £250. The idea of this technique is to focus daily on the sales opportunities that are waiting to be realized. No cold calling for us! Very important, you must write down your target and either keep it in your pocket or pin it up in the staff room. This will act as a constant reminder each moment of the day and it will keep your focus on sales.

A great idea is to have some pre-prepared cards kept on the reception desk. Each morning fill out your daily sales target. Below is an example, with point remind-ers I will explain following the chart.

Daily sales target sheet

1. People tend to buy from someone they like and trust	
DATE:	2. SALESPERSON:
TODAY'S DAILY TARGET IS:	£
3. SALES ACHIEVED	4. SALES REMAINING TO ACHIEVE
£ £ £ £ £ £	£ £ £ £ £ £

1 At the top of your daily sales target sheet write a statement to motivate or remind yourself of a selling principle that will help increase sales. Use a new fresh statement weekly or monthly. Other great ideas are:
   - 'Selling is taking the time to care about your clients' home-care.'
   - 'Whatever you focus on you tend to get more of.'
   - 'A smile … don't sell without it!'
   - 'If you don't close you don't sell.'
   - 'You will lose 100 per cent of the sales you don't ask for.'
   - 'Your clients are waiting for advice.'

2 Think Sales, feel Sales, act Sales. Write your name as a salesperson as oppose to a therapist.

3 Write down each sale as you achieve it.

4 Deduct it from your total so you see your sales remaining as achievable, this can be a great motivator as the day draws to a close.

You now have a target to work towards and you are no longer leaving your sales to chance. What you focus on you will get more of; focus on selling and your sales will increase. Look for those sales opportunities that are everywhere; for instance, when performing a manicure you could sell:

Manicure sales possibilities

Nail file	Nail varnish
Nail varnish remover	Nail hardener
Cuticle cream	Base coat
Nail oil	Top coat
Hand cream	Hand/body exfoliator

During a manicure you could effectively sell ten products – how many do you normally retail? After each manicure (at some point during the next seven to ten days) your clients will need to remove the varnish you have applied. Unless they have re-booked their treatments they will have to purchase a varnish remover from somewhere, make sure it is from your salon.

Keep focused at work, your clients love to be given advice on home-care from a true professional. During all your treatments give as much advice to your clients as you can, educate your clients on home-care, turn each appointment into a mini beauty school and keep focused. Ask yourself, 'Why has this client come to me?' Whilst I fully agree with the teaching model 'Don't be best friends with your clients', perhaps we have moved on since then. As we focus on relationship selling, the balance between friend and therapist is vital. You need a friendly approach with a professional touch.

The benefits of setting daily targets are:

- you begin each day with the right positive frame of mind

- it will keep you focused every day on sales opportunities

- it keeps you motivated as each target is achievable and realistic

- it makes you realize your sales potential

- each day is a new day, a new opportunity for success, you start afresh, motivated and determined to sell.

As a rule it takes a minimum of seven days of consistent action to create a habit. Spend at least 7–14 days setting daily targets and then move on to weekly targets.

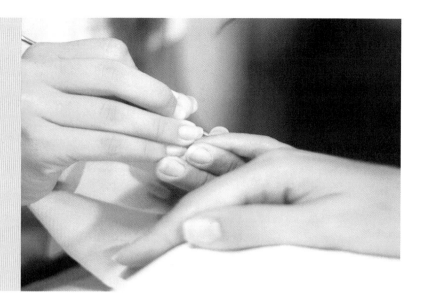

There are ten different products you could sell during a manicure – how many do you normally retail?

Setting weekly targets

Beginning with weekly targets is not always beneficial for everyone for two reasons. Firstly, if the weekly target is too low and you reach it within the first two days it can have a negative impact on your subconscious mind. Your mind could be sending a message saying: 'I have already achieved my target and can now just sit back for the rest of the week.' Secondly, if your weekly target is too high and your sales over the first two days are extremely low, your subconscious will be saying, this target is impossible to reach, so you could almost stop trying to sell.

After two weeks of setting daily targets, weekly targets can now be set for the following reasons:

- you will now look for sales opportunities each and every day

- you now know your capabilities and levels of sales that you can achieve on a daily basis

- if you have a low sales day through past experience you will have gathered an optimism that the rest of the week your sales can be high, therefore you will not lose motivation.

Set a weekly target that is realistic but also requires you to focus on selling and stretch your abilities that little bit further.

Initially to set yourself a weekly target just follow this simple formula:

1 Add together all your daily sales over the past two weeks, e.g. £1,000.

2 Divide this amount by two, e.g. £500.

Over the past two weeks your average weekly sales have been £500, now how much can you increase this by – 10 per cent, 20 per cent or how about 50 per cent?

Look how busy you are over the next week, what treatment mix is there in your column? Are there any new clients or clients requiring consultations? Add extra time to each facial treatment to give you the time to recommend products. All these points will help you create your weekly target.

Setting monthly targets

Moving on to monthly targets gives you a great opportunity to control your sales. At the beginning of each month you could invite a selection of clients for a complementary mini treatment and home-care advice or hold a beauty school. Brainstorm as many ideas to help accelerate your monthly sales and create the sales opportunities. This longer-term goal of monthly targets allows you time to work towards your sales goals and change your treatment mix.

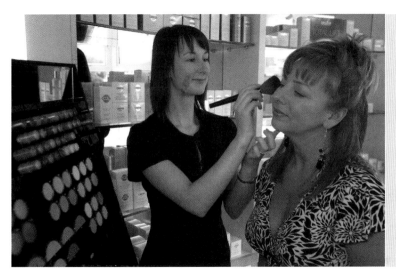

Planning events throughout the year will help you meet your regular sales targets

For some therapists weekly goals work best where others prefer monthly targets, choose what is right for you, but throughout the year plan events which will help increase sales and your opportunity to sell.

real life example

beautiful selling – my dream

Writing this book began as a dream; my vision was to be able to use my years of experience to help therapists retail both confidently and comfortably. My vision was to write a book that was both beneficial and useful. The art of selling is one that that I am not only passionate about, but also experienced and knowledgeable in. It is a skill I perform on a daily basis: I live the subject of retailing beauty products.

My dream became my goal and this book is the result.

> **dream big and you will achieve your goals**

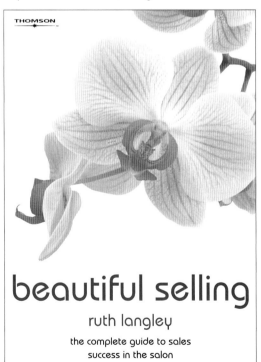

THOMSON

beautiful selling

ruth langley

the complete guide to sales
success in the salon

✔ **key** reminders

- Targets and goals are excellent motivators.
- Begin with daily targets, then progress to weekly and monthly targets.
- Look for sales opportunities each day – they are waiting to be found.
- Setting retail targets will keep you focused on selling.

Exercises

Make a copy of the daily sales target sheet. Each day for the next week create a daily sales target to achieve. At the end of the week observe how well you performed:

- How many sales did you create?
- Did you keep focused each and every day?
- Are your targets realistic?

Repeat this process for at least two weeks then move on to weekly targets.

Whatever you focus on in life you get more of. Try focusing on selling

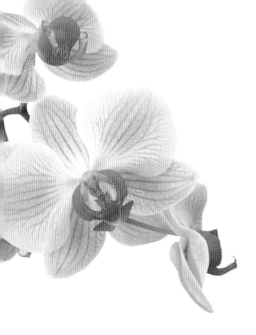

chapter 13
creating a sales culture in the salon

Introduction

Successful salon retailing is achieved through a concerted team effort. If you are a salon owner or manager it is your responsibility to keep your team focused on retail sales by being proactive. This chapter is devoted to areas that, as a sales manager (yes, you now have a new title), gives you the opportunity of having a positive impact. The growth of retail sales requires many ingredients such as time and training, but above all it is essential that all your team buy into your sales culture. The more serious you are about selling the more serious your team will be. Turn your attention to your team's sales levels and encourage them to approach selling in a positive result-orientated way.

you will learn

Within this chapter we will review:

- The importance of developing a positive sales environment
- How to understand your role as the sales manager
- How to introduce sales games, meetings and incentives to encourage your team

Relevant Habia modules for NVQ students: Unit G11

Some ideas and techniques

I have selected some ideas and techniques to help you with your new role as the salon's new sales manager.

Create a salon shop

Regardless of space a well-stocked salon shop will strengthen your identity. It creates awareness of your products and begins to help plant a seed that can develop a desire to buy.

The retail units should be:

- Fully stocked – this sends the correct message to your customers – we are passionate and firm believers in what we sell. Your clients will see that you have invested in the products. Good stock control is vital, as a salesperson the most disheartening feeling is when clients come to purchase a product and you realize you have none in stock.

- Positioned in the reception area so your clients feel comfortable to browse.

The products should be:

- Accessible – your clients should be able to touch and pick up the products.

- Priced – I believe all products should be clearly priced.

- Positioned – mainly between eye and knee level.

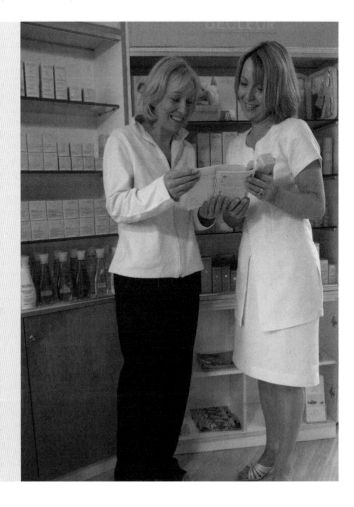

A well-stocked salon shop will strengthen your identity and build awareness of your products

- Merchandised – display your products soldier style so clients feel comfortable removing them. Soldier lines march out of the door, pretty displays stay pretty on the shelf.

Utilize key area such as the reception desk and coffee table for impulse buys. As much as a vase of flowers looks great on the reception desk we are not florists: devote this valuable space to retail sales.

Retail incentives

Commission

As a salon owner I believe that what gets rewarded gets repeated and feel paying commission to your therapists is essential. I understand that money is not the only motivator, indeed you will later read about other great incentives to offer your team. However, I believe money does suddenly become a motivator if you take it away. We all need financial security and the opportunity to increase our wealth. Offering a financial reward to your therapists each time they sell a product will increase their desire to help their clients buy products. It should obviously not be the only reason they sell but it will come into the equation. A flat rate of 10 per cent commission on sales seems to be the norm and can work quite well. However, I prefer to offer a three-tier commission structure of 5 per cent, 10 per cent and 15 per cent according to the level of sales achieved. If a therapist reaches weekly sales of over £600 she is really working hard for each sale and I believe in rewarding well for all her hard work: offering 15 per cent is a real motivator.

team incentives

Together

Everyone

Achieves

More

Team incentives

Getting the team to work together towards a sales target can be incredibly successful. Try and link the sales drive to a forthcoming event, such as celebrating the salon's anniversary. I annually treat my girls to an evening at the Doncaster races. Although I pay for the meal and entrance fee, I only put a set amount of money in the kitty for champagne and drinks. However, I realized this could be an area to offer a great sales incentive. I explained to my team that during the week leading up to our evening out, I would put 10 per cent of the total amount of retail sales into the drinks kitty. I called this incentive 'race for sales' and it was a huge success. It created fun, encouraged teamwork, increased sales and got the whole team focusing on retail. Needless to say, this incentive, as with the Doncaster races, has now become a permanent fixture.

As a salon manager try to constantly think of new ways to reward your team for their efforts.

Christmas is a time when spending on retail increases, so launch a special incentive scheme and offer your products or gift voucher for a local store as added incentives.

Fun days

Fun days are just that. I believe selling should be fun. Periodically just before we open the salon I announce that the team member who sells the most products during the day will receive a prize. The prize is usually a skin-care travel kit or a body product we retail or simply a £10 note in an envelope. This is a very short-term incentive which:

- boosts sales

- creates so much fun and laughter – great for team spirit

- jogs everybody's motivation back and gets the team to focus on giving their clients advice on retail products

The essence is just to enjoy and the winner is announced at the end of the day when they receive their prize.

A word of caution

Apart from fun days I never encourage competition between the therapists for several reasons.

- A new inexperienced therapist will initially be building her clientele and may not have the sales opportunities available yet.

- If a therapist has really worked hard and is just pipped at the post she may feel very demotivated.

- Some of my therapists work part-time and again may not have the same volume of sales opportunities.

There is a much more productive way to set targets to achieve great sales results and keep all team members focused and encouraged.

Setting personal targets

Take each individual therapist's sales figures for the past six weeks and divide by six to get their average weekly sales. Next set four targets for them personally to reach. Each stage once achieved receives a reward, again I use the salon retail products. I create a chart with all the therapists' names and targets printed on it

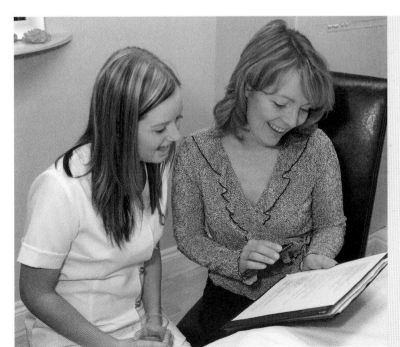

Creating an individualized sales target chart for your salon is a good way to motivate staff

and place it in the staff room. The girls then fill in their sales as they achieve them. This really creates excitement and anticipation particularly when they are close to reaching each target. However, although all the team can see how everyone is doing, their primary concern is their own performance. Observing other therapists' columns only acts as encouragement. Each week your therapists should be working towards their own personal target.

The above system is great to run fortnightly a few times a year for example at Christmas or during the summer.

 tip

- Do not be afraid to ask you skin-care supplier to send you some complementary retail products for you to use as team incentives.

- Explain that you are developing and growing the salon's retail sales and would really appreciate their support.

Retail training in department stores

A really effective training concept is to periodically (as a team) visit a department store and each team member pose as a customer who is looking for a new skin-care programme to use at home. The three benefits and results of this are:

1 You will know how it feels to be the customer. I believe the best way to teach customer care is to experience it and the same is true of selling. By becoming the customer you will experience how the sales process feels and this will have a major impact on your selling style.

2 You will learn their selling techniques. Some will be amazing, some good and some not so good, but each salesperson will hopefully have at least one new idea which can inspire you. This technique can then be taken back to the salon and implemented.

3 It is great fun. As we arrive at our chosen store we find the coffee shop and I sit and wait for each team member to return. One therapist will usually arrive back within a few minutes, whilst others may be gone for about 40

minutes. When all the team arrive back they share their experiences with the rest of the team and we all learn from each other. As you can imagine the team have a story to tell and we can guarantee laughter but also learning.

Sales games

Retail rollover

I believe learning should be fun so I created a sales game called 'Retail Rollover' that encapsulates the essence of selling – learning, teaching, asking questions, listening and enjoying the process.

How Retail Rollover works:

- Each team member is given the handout Retail Rollover (see below) one week prior to the sales meeting. Each therapist answers the questions and presents it to their fellow team members at the meeting.

- After the presentation the rest of the team ask questions about the product and or its uses.

- The results – all the team will learn a lot about the products being presented plus hear how the therapist recommends the product.

- At the end, place all the products in a group and each therapist has to decide which product they would purchase based entirely on the presentation. The product with the most votes wins and the therapist who gave the presentation wins the prize.

retail rollover handout

The idea for this concept is to empower, educate and motivate your fellow team members. You will be asked to present your answers and host a question and answer session within a five minute allocation time.

Please answer the following two questions to prepare for your winning presentation.

> ### question one
> What is your favourite retail product and why?
>
> ### question two
> How do you recommend this product to clients? Please include two ingredients and two benefits and the results you will receive from using the product.

At the end of retail rollover, the team member who has given the most effective presentation will win a prize.

Retail Rollover is simple, fun yet very effective. It is also amazing how the products that were demonstrated will suddenly see an increase in their level of sales.

Retail rollover extra

As an added bonus you will be able to observe your therapists' individual sales style. You can praise their good points but also make notes on areas which could be improved and consequently discuss them at their next individual meeting.

Retail Rollover is a tool which can be used again and again. The more it is used the more confident your therapists will become and the better their sales will be.

Sales training

The key to any training is to be consistent. Offer training to your team on a regular basis. Train your team on techniques and product knowledge and encourage them to share their sales experiences. The product information chart we discussed in Chapter 7 on product knowledge can be a great focal point to start your sales training, as it encourages all your therapists to learn about the products and their results.

Sales meetings

Each month devote a little time to spend with each team member to discuss their sales performance. Something I hear time and time again from salon owners is 'my therapists won't sell or don't sell'. Usually the real reason is they can't sell. They are unsure and have no confidence. As their sales manager it is essential you offer the support and advice to help them learn and develop this new skill.

Retail mission statement

Creating a retail mission statement will help develop a positive sales culture within your salon. Many salons will have a general mission statement saying what their business stands for. I took this idea and developed a retail mission statement that shows our strong passion for selling. By developing your own, you will demonstrate to your team that you are focused and determined to constantly achieve high retail sales. Below is a selection of ideas, but please develop one that is right for you, your team and your business.

retailing mission statement

- We have to provide our clients with the best home-care advice – this is our duty.
- The products we recommend must be the right choice for our clients and deliver results.
- Our clients have to be happy with their purchases.
- At the centre of every sale are our clients – never forget this.
- If we serve well we will sell well.
- Confidence comes from knowing that we can provide the best solution for our clients' concerns.

After you and your team have developed the mission statement ensure a copy is placed in the team room. Another good idea is to print small credit-card sizes of the mission statement, laminate them and give one to each team member.

Start the day in a 'selling way'

To empower your team, try holding a five-minute meeting just before opening the salon. This five-minute power talk can cover any area of the sales process that will encourage and motivate your team and help them focus on retail. You could discuss the importance of building relationships, selling the benefits or absolutely anything that will help your team. Try using motivational quotes that will inspire your therapists. Remember: the teacher learns most, so encourage a team member to host the meeting.

 real life example

lead by example

As a salon owner I have many roles and responsibilities to the salon, the clients and the team. I still, however, work on the salon floor as a beauty therapist and I am privileged to be able to do this.

As salon owners and managers we should lead by example in all areas of salon life and this should be apparent in selling.

I recently received a compliment from my receptionist; she was observing me selling to a client in reception. After the client had left the salon she said: 'I love watching you sell, I could watch you for hours.'

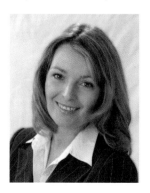

I do deliberately sell in front of my team and share my sales experiences with them.

Selling is a service that I promote as normal and natural within the salon.

Recently we employed a young girl to help out with general salon duties. She is still at school and just helps out at the weekend and some evenings after school. During a sales incentive I was running in the salon all the team members were required to record their sales on a chart in the team room. One afternoon I was looking at their sales figures and noticed this young girl had added her name and wrote down her achievements. At the tender age of 16 she was not only selling but she was proud of it!

✔ key reminders

- As the salon manager you need to help your team focus on sales. Lead by example.

- Ensure your salon shop is well stocked and change product displays regularly.

- Remember, what gets rewarded gets repeated. Offer individual commission schemes and team targets to encourage selling.

- Hold sales training and meetings to motivate, monitor and encourage your team.

Exercises

1 A well-stocked and well-displayed salon shop sends a powerful message to your clients: we believe in our products. Observe your retail displays. Following the advice in this chapter, what improvements can you make?

2 If you are the salon owner now is the time to begin some sales training:

   a Copy the Retail Rollover handout.
   b Distribute to each team member with guidelines on how to fill it in.
   c Plan a mini meeting (30 minutes) and observe the results.

A great idea is to do Retail Rollover every week. The more you play this sales game, the better and more confident your therapists will become. You could use this tool each day as part of your morning 'power talk'.

Whatever your faith ...
believe in yourself

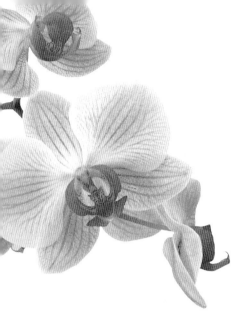

chapter fourteen
...and finally

Effective, beautiful selling

With the rapid growth in the skin-care industry, now is an exciting time to discover and develop your sales potential. As a professional and experienced therapist you are perfectly qualified to offer the best product advice and home-care recommendations to your clients. Direct your focus and take your sales to the next level. It will not always be easy and at times may seem overwhelming. The key is to keep going, never quit.

I am regularly asked 'What makes a therapist good at selling?' or 'What is the one thing that will increase my retail sales?' The truth is it is a combination of factors. As I have previously said, there is no magic formula to selling, just the application of proven techniques that begin the moment your clients enter the salon.

... consistently take action

Take small steps each and every day towards your sales target. Your success is down to you. Take control, use this book as a reference guide and keep applying its principles.

... remember

You already have many qualities and skills that are required to be effective at selling. Focus on relationships, put your clients first and offer a service second to none.

... and in conclusion

As I write the conclusion to *Beautiful Selling* I have to recall a sales scenario which happened just two days ago. A client, to whom I had given some samples to a few weeks ago, was sitting in the reception waiting for her therapist. I asked her if she had enjoyed trying the products and she commented how good they were and could she have some more information about them. As I began to sell, two more clients entered the salon and sat next to us. What followed is the essence of selling; as I began talking and demonstrating all three clients joined in. It became a fun selling experience, I was entertaining the clients. Each client tried the products, gave their positive feedback and were really enjoying the whole experience:

- I had an audience

- I was entertaining them

- I was making selling fun

- Buying then became fun.

You may have many reasons for not achieving your sales potential, for example:

- I do not have time to sell, or

- My clients buy from a local store where they receive bonus points every time they buy.

These reasons may be valid but the truth is we all have situations that could potentially limit us, the question is do we let them? The answer is no.

> ## remember always sell with passion

You have the potential to become a successful salesperson and I believe you will.

Enjoy selling beautifully!

Ruth

xxx

Clients love to be sold
to by a true
professional

index